RHEUMATISM AND MUSCULOSKELETAL DISORDERS

KYPHOSIS

CAUSES, METHODS OF TREATMENT AND POTENTIAL COMPLICATIONS

RHEUMATISM AND MUSCULOSKELETAL DISORDERS

Additional books in this series can be found on Nova's website under the Series tab.

Additional e-books in this series can be found on Nova's website under the e-book tab.

RHEUMATISM AND MUSCULOSKELETAL DISORDERS

KYPHOSIS

CAUSES, METHODS OF TREATMENT AND POTENTIAL COMPLICATIONS

JANICE NEWTON
EDITOR

New York

Library of Congress Cataloging-in-Publication Data

ISBN: 978-1-63483-224-3
Library of Congress Control Number: 2015943275

Published by Nova Science Publishers, Inc. † New York

Contents

Preface

Kyphosis is an abnormal increased forward angulation of the spine which results in a minimal to severe spinal deformity producing a slouching posture. Patients may present with progressive deformity accompanied by associated consequences including neck pain, neurologic dysfunction, postural instability, and marked decline in health-related quality of life. This book discusses what may be the cause of kyphosis, the methods of treatment available and other potential complications it leads to.

Chapter I – Classification of kyphosis based upon the clinical presentation, regional involvement, severity and various etiological causes is described.

Chapter II – Early-onset scoliosis (EOS) is defined as scoliosis diagnosed before age 10. Not only do these patients have spinal deformity, they may also have thoracic malformations, such as fused or absent ribs. Early-onset scoliosis is uncommon, however it is an important health issue because, if left untreated, is at risk for rapid deformity progression, pulmonary insufficiency and possibly early mortality. In healthy children, there is a tendency for thoracic kyphosis, lumbar lordosis, pelvic incidence and pelvic tilt to increase with age, while sacral slope usually remains relatively stable. Children with scoliosis show somewhat similar pelvic incidence, but have higher pelvic tilt and lower sacral slope values as compared to healthy children. Treatment options for EOS include observation, bracing, casting, and surgery depending on age and severity of the curvature. Spinal fusion is generally not recommended as an initial treatment in skeletally immature patients, as it will effectively stop the growth of the child's spine, chest wall, and pulmonary system. As a result, the most common surgical treatments for early-onset scoliosis are growth friendly surgeries, such as spinal growing rods or vertical expandable prosthetic titanium ribs (VEPTR). These growth friendly devices permit continued spine growth, maximize the space available for the lung, and are thought to enhance pulmonary function. Proximal junctional kyphosis (PJK) is a non-physiologic, sagittal plane angulation that occurs cephalad to an instrumented spine. In adults, proximal junctional failures above deformity constructs have been well established with different risk factors identified; however, the incidence and nature of this kyphosis remains unclear. In young children, this deformity has only recently been described for growth friendly techniques. So far, there has been no consensus on one definition for this deformity with different angles and measurement levels being described in the literature, which range from 6% to 56% incidence of PJK. Sagittal spinopelvic parameters may help predict the risk of PJK for this population, with higher rates found in older children who are hyper-kyphotic pre-operatively and in those who have positive post-operative sagittal balance. Ultimately, PJK is a radiographic parameter. The authors believe that it may be also predispose to implant failure and to the choice of upper instrumented level during revision or graduate surgery. Indications for revision surgery include a deformity sufficiently severe to endanger the neural elements, or the concern that a further increase in the deformity would necessitate a far more difficult revision technique. Revision surgeries included revising the failed implant (rods) to include more cephalad vertebrae, revising VEPTRs into growing rods and definitive fusion techniques. Further studies should be performed to determine what amount of PJK may be predictive of these clinically relevant complications and the need for surgical intervention.

Chapter III – Kyphosis is the most common spinal deformity of the cervical spine. Patients may present with progressive deformity and adverse associated consequences, including neck pain, neurologic dysfunction, postural instability, and a marked decline in health-related quality of life. As patients develop further progression of kyphosis, neck pain, inability to achieve horizontal gaze, and neurological deficits may worsen due to a combination of nerve root or spinal cord traction. In this circumstance, surgical correction of kyphosis has been shown to have the most pivotal role in improving clinical results. Although many patients with cervical kyphosis (CK) present with similar complaints, numerous etiologies have been reported, including trauma, neoplasm, post-radiation, degenerative disease, systemic arthritides, neuromuscular disorders, infection, and iatrogenic conditions (e.g., following cervical laminectomy). Determining the specific cause is critical to appreciate the unique precautions and considerations that may influence the approach to treatment. A thorough, systematic clinical and radiographic evaluation of every patient is necessary to direct appropriate treatment, both non-operative and surgical. For relatively mild cases of cervical deformity without neurologic deficits, non-operative treatment with activity modification, physical therapy, or bracing can be considered. However, for severe, progressively worsening deformity with evidence of neurologic deficits, or chin-on-chest deformity affecting the ability to achieve horizontal gaze, surgical intervention is recommended. Although surgery may be performed by anterior, posterior, or combined approaches, the decision on which approach and, if necessary, a particular sequence of staged approaches is based on both patient-specific factors and surgeon preference. In general, kyphosis correction is obtained by lengthening the anterior column of the spine, shortening the posterior column of the spine, or a combination of both. Because of the proximity of the spinal cord, nerve roots, and vertebral arteries, it may be necessary to correct in multiple stages with several approaches. Many combinations of the above approaches have been described in the literature, each with their respective advantages and disadvantages, thus highlighting their differential utility given the patients' presenting condition. Due to the potentially extensive, prolonged nature of the surgical procedures, surgeons must be cognizant and anticipate for potential post-operative adjuncts to facilitate recovery and reduce complications, such as delayed extubation and consideration of placement of a feeding tube. Furthermore, anticipating potential complications and taking specific precautionary measures with careful pre-operative planning can help reduce the incidence of adverse events post-operatively. The treatment of patients with cervical kyphosis is challenging. Proper evaluation requires an appreciation of the various causes contributing to the deformity, a thorough understanding of the anatomical structures, and an appreciation of the surgical options available including the use of combined surgical approaches or complex correctional techniques to achieve optimal patient outcomes.

Chapter IV – Scheuermann's disease is a type of permanent structural kyphosis which develops in approximately 0.4 to 8.3% of the pre-adolescent population. The deformity is radiographically defined by the vertebral wedging of at least three adjacent vertebral bodies angled a minimum of 5°. The reported etiology and the incidence amongst sexes vary widely amongst studies. Scheuermann's kyphosis is histologically identified by the disorganized and defective endochondral ossification of vertebral end plates resulting in a disruption of growth. The biochemical dysbalance of the matrix components, collagen and mucopolysaccharide, render the vertebral end plate weak and vulnerable to mechanical strains, resulting in the pathognomonic vertebral wedging. Different hypotheses have been discussed as origins of the disorder. In fact, juvenile osteoporosis, the level of physical activity, weight and height, as well as sternum length and growth hormone levels have been discussed as potential contributing or causal factors of the disease. Great dissent in the scientific community exists to this day pertaining the degree of influence of genetics on the pathogenesis of the disease. Patients with Scheuermann's disease may present at a diverse range of age with complaints of pain, postural changes and rarely neurological or cardiopulmonary compromise. Upon clinical examination, patients will demonstrate excessive fixed kyphosis in the thoracic- or lumbar vertebrae with little or no correction on hyperextension. Non-structural compensatory features may also include pelvic anteversion, shoulder rounding and lumbar as well as cervical hyperlordosis. Radiographs of the spine demonstrate kyphotic deformity in the thoracic, thoracolumbar or lumbar vertebrae associated with vertebral wedging and disk space narrowing between the angulated vertebrae. Additional typical features which may be found are end plate irregularities and intraosseous disk herniations, also referred to as Schmorl nodes. The management of Scheuermann's disease has traditionally been focused on conservative measures such as observation, symptomatic pain relief, physical therapy and rehabilitation as well as bracing. The only relative indications for surgery have been failure of conservative measures resulting in progressive curvature and pain. Rarely, neurologic or cardiopulmonary compromise as well as unacceptable cosmesis may lead to the invasive correction of the kyphotic deformity. The long-term outcome studies comparing conservative versus surgical treatment measures have however demonstrated no difference in the outcome of the degree of kyphosis related to the method of treatment.

Chapter V – Kyphosis is a progressive, curvature of thoracic spine which results in rounding or bowing of the back . Curved spine accompanied by restricted neck motion and poor lung reserve present challenges for an ophthalmic surgeon who is used to patient's neck and head resting flat on the operating table and the eye in the horizontal position. Intraoperative difficulties include poor view, inability to maneuver surgical instruments properly and constant threat of elevated vitreous pressure. Several innovative solutions have been published including, maximal reverse Trendelenburg position with pillows under the head and neck, use of a donut and wedge shaped head positioner, allowing the patient to remain in upright sitting position while their head is positioned horizontally in a modified waiting room chair, performing surgery while standing, using 4-section orthopedic operating table, laying the patients on their sides, *side saddle* positioning, face-to-face positioning, parachute type harness inferior corneal retraction suture, or extreme patient positioning for retinal surgery. This chapter highlights various surgical options to facilitate surgeons pick the best course of action when dealing with intraocular surgery in patients with kyphosis.

Chapter VI – Non-Operative Treatments. Observation: Observation is usually the first method of treatment for a young child with a spinal deformity. The visits to the physician will be spaced according to the likelihood of measuring a significant change in the X-ray between each visit. Type I deformities are more likely to have several visits per year. Severe or progressive congenital kyphosis deformities greater than 45° or kyphosis associated with neurologic weakness are usually treated surgically. Early surgical intervention generally produces the best results and can halt progression of the curve. The type of surgical procedure will depend on the nature of the abnormality. Bracing: Unfortunately, bracing is not recommended when treating congenital scoliosis. Clinical studies fail to demonstrate improved patient outcomes with this method of treatment. Surgical Treatments. In Situ Fusion: The surgical choice for a progressive kyphotic deformity is a solid fusion or arthrodesis of the deformed vertebrae. The fusion may also include one normal vertebra above and one normal vertebra below this area. Bone graft from the patient or tissue bank is placed posteriorly, on the back of the spine, along the area of the abnormality. In severely angulated curves, additional bone graft may be placed anteriorly, on the front of the spine, as well as from behind. The fusion may be performed with or without the use of instrumentation. In situ fusion is a non-instrumented fusion without correction of the angulation. The bone graft will require 4-6 months to mature into a solid fusion mass. During the postoperative period the fusion must be protected with a cast or brace until X-rays demonstrate a solid fusion. Instrumented Fusion and Osteotomy. With progressive kyphotic curves in older children, surgery may include instrumentation (rods, hooks, and screws) that helps to correct the deformity. If the spinal cord is unable to tolerate the manipulative techniques that "straighten" the spine, the surgeon may consider the removal of the mis-shapened vertebrae to realign the spine. Pedicle subtraction osteotomies and Vertebral column resections are various methods of treatment depending upon severity of deformity and surgeon preference.

In: Kyphosis
Editor: Janice Newton

ISBN: 978-1-63483-224-3

Chapter I

Causes and Classification of Kyphosis

Kush Kumar, MD
Carl Vinson VA Medical Ctr., Dublin, GA, US

Abstract

Classification of kyphosis based upon the clinical presentation, regional involvement, severity and various etiological causes is described.

Kyphosis (from Greek κυφός kyphos, a hump) is the abnormally increased forward angulation of the spine. This results in a minimal to severe spinal deformity producing slouching posture. It can be limited to the cervical, thoracic, lumbar spinal regions or may involve multiple regions.

Kyphosis may be classified as generalized, involving a large segment of the spine, or localized, involving a limited segment of the spine. Generalized kyphosis usually produces a C-shaped deformity of the spine. Hence the layman term of 'hunchback" or "roundback." When the "roundness" of the upper spine is greater than 45° it is referred to as "humpback" or "hyperkyphosis." Localized kyphosis however demonstrates an angular or "V" shaped deformity.

Some common causes of generalized kyphosis include postural kyphosis, Scheuermann's disease, achondroplasia, Paget's disease, ankylosing spondylitis (Bechterew's disease), muscular dystrophy, poliomyelitis and osteoporosis. Generalized kyphosis may also occur as a consequence of a nutritional etiology and is noted primarily in the developing world. It often presents with vitamin D deficiency or rickets in children and osteomalacia in adults. Fluorosis is another but uncommon cause of kyphosis. The "Hunchback of Notre-Dame" or "Dowager's hump" is also a generalized kyphosis seen in the senile postmenopausal patients and is associated with the osteoporotic collapse of multiple vertebrae. Kyphosis involving larger segment of spine can also present during in the teenage years, commonly in children with neurological disorders such as cerebral palsy. Other causes of kyphosis include osteogenesis imperfecta, osteopetrosis (Albers-Schonberg disease), certain endocrine and connective tissue disorders. Osteoarthritis, renal osteodystrophy, inflammatory spondylosis and DISH syndrome may also produce kyphosis involving variable segments of the spine and result in a localized or generalized condition. Kyphosis in neurofibromatosis may be localized or generalized depending upon the extent of the spine involved.

Trauma, tumor, and tuberculosis of the spine are the most common conditions that lead to a localized kyphosis. Osteochondritis (Calvé's disease) of a vertebral body, also known as vertebra plana producing kyphotic deformity is often diagnosed radiologically. Kyphosis in tuberculosis of the spine, or Pott's disease, has been described as K1, or "knuckle" kyphus ($<10^0$), K2, or angular kyphus (11^0 to 60^0), and K3 ($>60^0$), or gibbus. K1 and K2 are the early and advanced stages of the disease respectively when collapse is limited to the adjacent two vertebrae. K1 is a palpable kyphus, noted during the clinical examination whereas K2 is a visible kyphus, producing obvious deformity. K3 is seen when a larger segment of spine consisting of multiple vertebrae are involved [1]. Prediction of the angle of gibbus deformity in children with tuberculosis of spine can also be made and calculated [2].

Kyphosis may also be subdivided into two categories, congenital and acquired. Congenital kyphosis is present at birth and occurs during fetal development due to improper segmentation of the spine during embryogenesis. Klippel–Feil deformity involves cervical spine and may be associated with other developmental anomalies. The VACTERL syndrome (abnormalities of the vertebrae, anus, cardiovascular tree, trachea, esophagus, renal system, and limb buds) is an extreme example of association of malformation in the embryonic stage. Spina Bifida (Latin: "split spine") and myelomeningocele may also be associated with congenital kyphosis. Vertebral error of segmentation may be due to malformation, disruption or deformation of the developing vertebral sclerotome.

Kyphoscoliosis is kyphosis associated with scoliosis and often seen in association with other congenital birth defects and other musculoskeletal disorders. It leads to asymmetric weakening of the paraspinal muscles causing chronic poor ventilation of the lungs. Progressive severe, kyphoscoliotic curvature of the spine may interfere with respiration. It may also lead to chronic pulmonary hypertension. Kyphoscoliosis may be seen in Duchenne muscular dystrophy, Friedreich's ataxia, Ehlers-Danlos syndrome, syringomyelia and spondyloepiphyseal dysplasia. Kyphoscoliosis noted in several such conditions have genetic basis. The lateral subluxation of the spine, a deformity rarely noted in Pott's disease, when both anterior and posterior elements of the vertebrae are involved, a "composite vertebral involvement" may also produce kyphoscoliosis [3].

References

[1] Kumar K, Tuberculosis of Spine - Natural History of Disease and its Judicious Management: *The J. of the Western Pacific Orthopedic Association.* Vol. XXV, No.1, 1-8, 1988.

[2] Rajasekaran S, and Shanmugasundram, TK. Prediction of the angle of gibbus deformity in tuberculosis of the spine. J Bone & Joint Surg, 69A:503-508,1987.

[3] Kumar K, *A Clinical Study of Posterior Spinal Tuberculosis and its Classification: International Orthopaedics* (SICOT) Vol. 9, No. 4, 147-152, 1985.

In: Kyphosis
Editor: Janice Newton

ISBN: 978-1-63483-224-3

Chapter II

Proximal Junctional Kyphosis in Early Onset Scoliosis

Ron El-Hawary*, MD, MSc, FRCS(C), and Mohamad S. Yasin, M.B,B.S

[1]Associate Professor of Surgery (Orthopaedics)
Associate Professor of Surgery (Neurosurgery)
Associate Professor School of Biomedical Engineering
Dalhousie University, Chief of Paediatric Orthopaedic Surgery
IWK Health Centre, Halifax, NS, Canada
[2]Fellow in Paediatric Orthopaedic Surgery,
IWK Health Centre, Halifax, NS, Canada

Abstract

Early-onset scoliosis (EOS) is defined as scoliosis diagnosed before age 10. Not only do these patients have spinal deformity, they may also have thoracic malformations, such as fused or absent ribs. Early-onset scoliosis is uncommon, however it is an important health issue because, if left untreated, is at risk for rapid deformity progression, pulmonary insufficiency and possibly early mortality. In healthy children, there is a tendency for thoracic kyphosis, lumbar lordosis, pelvic incidence and

* Email: ron.el-hawary@iwk.nshealth.ca.

pelvic tilt to increase with age, while sacral slope usually remains relatively stable. Children with scoliosis show somewhat similar pelvic incidence, but have higher pelvic tilt and lower sacral slope values as compared to healthy children.

Treatment options for EOS include observation, bracing, casting, and surgery depending on age and severity of the curvature. Spinal fusion is generally not recommended as an initial treatment in skeletally immature patients, as it will effectively stop the growth of the child's spine, chest wall, and pulmonary system. As a result, the most common surgical treatments for early-onset scoliosis are growth friendly surgeries, such as spinal growing rods or vertical expandable prosthetic titanium ribs (VEPTR). These growth friendly devices permit continued spine growth, maximize the space available for the lung, and are thought to enhance pulmonary function.

Proximal junctional kyphosis (PJK) is a non-physiologic, sagittal plane angulation that occurs cephalad to an instrumented spine. In adults, proximal junctional failures above deformity constructs have been well established with different risk factors identified; however, the incidence and nature of this kyphosis remains unclear.

In young children, this deformity has only recently been described for growth friendly techniques. So far, there has been no consensus on one definition for this deformity with different angles and measurement levels being described in the literature, which range from 6% to 56% incidence of PJK. Sagittal spinopelvic parameters may help predict the risk of PJK for this population, with higher rates found in older children who are hyper-kyphotic pre-operatively and in those who have positive post-operative sagittal balance. Ultimately, PJK is a radiographic parameter. We believe that it may be also predispose to implant failure and to the choice of upper instrumented level during revision or graduate surgery. Indications for revision surgery include a deformity sufficiently severe to endanger the neural elements, or the concern that a further increase in the deformity would necessitate a far more difficult revision technique. Revision surgeries included revising the failed implant (rods) to include more cephalad vertebrae, revising VEPTRs into growing rods and definitive fusion techniques. Further studies should be performed to determine what amount of PJK may be predictive of these clinically relevant complications and the need for surgical intervention.

Early Onset Scoliosis

James et al., in 1954, categorized idiopathic scoliosis according to the age of onset into: infantile, presenting before 3 years of age; juvenile between 4 and 9 years; and adolescent appearing from age 10 years until the end of growth [1]. This classification was thought to correlate with periods of increased growth velocity, however, during the juvenile period spinal growth decelerates and scoliosis onset is uncommon [2]. Spinal growth usually parallels that of the chest wall and lung parenchyma. While two thirds of the final sitting height is achieved by age 5 years [2], thoracic volume reaches around 30% of adult volume by age 5 years and 50% by age 10 years. In addition, The number of pulmonary alveoli increases about 10 folds during growth, primarily during the first 8 years of life [3].

Given the importance of the first few years in life in coupling spinal and thoracic cavity growth, the classification of scoliosis into early and late onset was made. Early-onset scoliosis (EOS) is defined as "scoliosis with onset less than the age of ten years, regardless of etiology." This definition does not only include idiopathic etiologies, but also congenital, neuromuscular and syndromic ones [4]. Not only do these patients have spinal deformity, they may also have thoracic malformations, such as fused or absent ribs. An increasing body of evidence suggests that patients in whom scoliosis develops at an early age, regardless of the cause, are at significant risk for thoracic insufficiency syndrome, defined as an inability of the thorax to support normal respiration and lung growth [5]. Early-onset scoliosis remains uncommon, however it is an important health issue because, if left untreated, is at risk for rapid deformity progression, pulmonary insufficiency and possibly early mortality. In 1959 James et al. [6] described progressive early onset scoliosis as one that "develops rapidly and relentlessly, causing the severest form of orthopedic cripple with dreadful deformity, marked dwarfing and shortening of life."

It has been clearly demonstrated in the literature that one of the aims of management in patients with scoliosis is to improve or maintain their overall coronal and sagittal balance. Although sagittal spinopelvic parameters and their natural history during the first 10 years of life have been defined for normal children [7], it has not been until recently that these parameters have been defined for young children with scoliosis and compared with their normal peers. In healthy children, there is a tendency for thoracic kyphosis, lumbar lordosis, pelvic incidence and pelvic tilt to increase with age, while sacral slope usually remains relatively stable [8]. C7 plumb line tends to move posterior from childhood to adulthood and is normally seen intersecting the posterior superior corner of the first sacral vertebral body, but its progressive forward displacement should raise a suspicion for the risk of developing spinal pathology [8]. In a recent study be El-Hawary et al. [9], 80 patients with early onset scoliosis of various etiologies were evaluated for sagittal balance, thoracic kyphosis, lumbar lordosis, pelvic incidence, pelvic tilt, sacral slope, and pelvic radius angle. These baseline parameters were compared with normal values from previous reports. He concluded that children with scoliosis show somewhat similar pelvic incidence, but have higher pelvic tilt and lower sacral slope values as compared to healthy children. Results of all these studies should be directed toward aiding surgeons in trying to restore abnormal parameters to normal values, as failure to do so with resultant sagittal imbalance may have deleterious effects on the future of these children.

Natural History and Treatment of Early Onset Scoliosis

The natural history of EOS is one of severe progressive deformity, restrictive-type lung disease, cardiac diseases and increased mortality. Conclusive evidence that treatment improves this natural history is lacking [10], a fact possibly explained by the rarity of the condition and the difficulty of performing lifetime-long follow up studies. However as for all other types of scoliosis, the management of every patient with early onset scoliosis shall remain individualized, even though challenging. Taking into consideration the age, underlying pathology, severity, progression potential, associated conditions, and of course family preference if applicable; the management options have greatly varied. Starting with observation, to bracing, casting, and surgery, all are valid modalities of treatment in order of invasiveness.

Derotational serial casting, with routine cast changes every 2-4 months, is currently indicated for progressive curves with Cobb angle between 25 and 60 degrees, and for curves with anticipated progression (rib vertebral angle difference > 20 degrees and/or rib phase 2).

Traditional fusion surgery to control scoliosis progression has several negative effects: Cessation of spinal growth, reduction in ultimate spine height, deleterious effects on chest wall growth, thoracic insufficiency syndrome and crankshaft. The effect of fusion surgery on forced vital capacity (FVC) was shown by Goldberg et al. [10], where patients fused younger than ten years of age had FVC of 41% of the normal at maturity, compared to 68% for patients fused after ten years. And because vital capacity less than 43% of the predicted normal value is considered a risk factor for respiratory failure [11], these patients have a guarded prognosis for long-term pulmonary function. As a result, there has been a paradigm shift in the last decade towards growth friendly surgeries. This philosophy is that there is more focus on the growth of the spine, lung and chest wall rather than just achieving a short straight spine. Fusion surgery is now seen as a last resort.

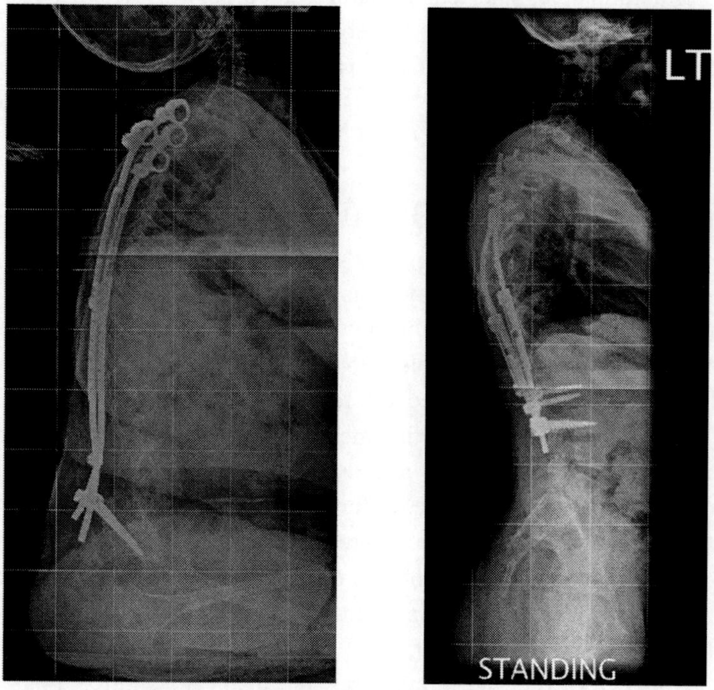

(a) (b)

Figure 1. Examples of posterior distraction based growth friendly implants. (a) Lateral radiograph of a Rib-based distraction system (VEPTR) in a patient with neuromuscular early onset scoliosis (cerebral palsy). (b) Lateral radiograph of a spine-based distraction system in a patient with syndromic early onset scoliosis (Goldenhar syndrome).

Attempting to delay the need for definitive surgery until after 10 years of age, in order to allow for appropriate spine and thoracic growth is the goal of the growth friendly principle of scoliosis surgery. Skaggs et al. [12] described a classification system of growth friendly spinal implants to allow researchers and clinicians to have a common language and facilitate comparative studies. He categorized growth friendly spinal implants into 3 major systems: Distraction-based systems; correcting deformities by applying distractive forces across deformed segments with anchors at the top and bottom of the system attached to the spine, rib and/or pelvis [13]. Examples include spine or rib-based single or dual growing rods, vertical expandable prosthetic titanium ribs (VEPTR; Depuy Synthes Spine, Raynham, MA), and remotely expandable devices (Figure 1). Compression-based systems; applying compressive forces to the curve convexity causing growth inhibition, and they include vertebral staples and tethers. And guided growth systems; correcting deformities by anchoring multiple vertebrae including apical ones with initial translational corrective forces, and these include Luque trolley and Shilla (Medtronic Spine, Memphis, TN).

Complications of Growth Friendly Surgery

The use of Distraction based systems has led to an overall improvement in Cobb angle and in spine length; however, patients are still faced with increased spine stiffness, possible worsening of the rotational deformity (crankshaft), auto fusion, the need for routine lengthening surgeries every 6 months, and most importantly inconclusive pulmonary outcome as the increased forced vital capacity is usually coupled with decreased respiratory compliance and increased thoracic stiffness [14]. Compressive systems on the other hand take advantage of the Hueter-Volkmann law applicability to the spine [15] with the potential advantages of being reversible and a single event surgery. However; overcorrection and limiting spine growth in a young patient may still not be ideal. As for the guided growth techniques; potential benefits include avoidance of repeated procedures, but again the shortcomings of less growth and auto-fusion still exist.

Sankar et al. [16] compared complications rate in 36 children with early onset spinal deformity treated with various types of growth friendly implants by a single surgeon. The implants included dual rod spine-based distraction, rib-based distraction, and hybrid constructs with rib anchors proximally and spine anchors distally. An overall uniformly high complication rate of 2.06 per patient was found. Even though there was a trend toward fewer complications in hybrid constructs, he was not able to demonstrate a statistically significant difference among the three implant types in terms of the number of complications.

Bess and colleagues [17] analyzed one hundred and forty patients with EOS treated with growing rods from the multicentre growing spine study group database with a minimum follow up of two years. 58% had at least one complication, with 27% of patients with single rods required unplanned procedures in comparison to 10% of the two rods population. To reduce the risk of complications, they suggested to delay initial implantation of the growing rods if possible and to limit the number of lengthening procedure. Another multicenter study from Japan by Watanabe et al. [18] assessed the risk factors associated with growing rod surgery for EOS. He reviewed 88 patients from 12 centers and found that complications affected 57% of the patients, significant independent risk factors included; an increase of every 20° in the proximal thoracic Cobb angle, an increase of every 20° in the thoracic kyphosis angle, and 6 or more rod lengthening procedures.

Lucas and colleagues [19] reviewed the French experience of complications in EOS patients treated with VEPTRs. In their series 54 patients with 184 total procedures had a complication rate of 137% per patient and 40% per surgery, and only 4 patients developed static disturbances in their sagittal plane. Schroerlucke et al. [20] conducted a retrospective review of a multicenter series and concluded that patients with EOS with higher than normal thoracic kyphosis prior to growing rod surgery had significantly more general and implant-related complications than patients with normal thoracic kyphosis. Implant complications included anchor failure, prominent implant, and most commonly rod breakage.

Proximal Junctional Kyphosis - General

Proximal junctional kyphosis (PJK) is a non-physiologic, sagittal plane angulation that occurs cephalad to an instrumented spine.

In adults and adolescents, proximal junctional failures above deformity constructs have been well established with different risk factors identified; however, the incidence, nature and clinical significance of this kyphosis remains unclear. Several reports in the literature have shed light on PJK in adults and adolescents with variable definition, incidence, prevalence, risk factors, clinical significance and the need for revision surgery. Moreover, it followed diverse primary pathologies treated with different surgical techniques using variable types of fusion instrumentation.

The most consistent Proximal junctional angle measurement in the literature as outlined by Glattes et al. [21] has been defined between the caudal endplate of the upper instrumented vertebra (UIV) and the cephalad endplate of 2 levels above the UIV, with abnormal PJK defined as having proximal junctional Cobb angle ≥ +10° and at least 10° greater than the pre-operative measurement [22-31]. Despite this consensus, there will always be difficulty in interpreting radiographic studies as to the effect of arm and head position on lateral radiographs, especially when evaluating the C7-T2 junction [22]. That's why Carmen et al. [32] considered that a change in a kyphosis measurement should be >10° to be 95% confident that the change is true.

Kim et al. [33] conducted a systematic review on PJK after spinal deformity fusion surgery. He was able to include 7 studies [22, 26-31] according to his selection criteria, all sharing the aforementioned definition. He reported a PJK incidence of 17%-39% mostly noted by 2 years postoperative with a moderate level of evidence. Risk factors of significance identified included; increased age, fusion to sacrum, combined anterior and posterior spinal fusion, thoracoplasty, UIV at T1–T3, and nonanatomic restoration of thoracic kyphosis. The type of instrument used at the proximal level (hooks, wires, or pedicle screws) did not have a consistent statistically significant association with PJK across studies. He also concluded that PJK does not seem to have a detrimental effect on health related quality of life (HRQOL) outcomes, at least in milder/non-revision forms. Glattes et al. [21] and Kim et al. [26] also showed that there were no significant differences in Scoliosis Research Society Patient Questionnaire-24 outcome-scores between the PJK and non-PJK group in their series.

Hostin et al. [34] reported a low PJK incidence of 5.6% with a variable definition including UIV fracture or the need for proximal extension of fusion, and at the two year mark Lee et al. [35] was able to report a 46% PJK prevalence.

Other risk factors reported in the literature include; male gender [26], segmental posterior instrumentation [25, 29, 37], pre-existing low bone mineral density and greater sagittal vertical axis change [24], pre-existing thoracic kyphosis more than 30° [23], stopping fusion at T3 in the upper thoracic spine [21], disruption of the posterior ligamentous complex during posterior fusion [21, 24, 28, 29, 35, 36], the use of intra-operative distraction [29, 38], the number of fused levels [39], use of pedicle screws [26, 29, 36], and the use of hybrid fixation [22].

Proximal Junctional Kyphosis in Early Onset Scoliosis

Proximal Junctional Kyphosis in early onset scoliosis treated with growth friendly techniques has only been recently described, and thus still there is no consensus on the definition, angles and measurement used, and the true incidence. PJK risk from 7% to 56% was reported in three studies from 2011 in the literature [40, 41, 42]. As those studies were performed on different samples of young patients with scoliosis and used three different definitions of PJK, it is unclear as to whether the differences in observed risk were related to the different patient samples examined in those studies or to the choice of PJK definition that was used. Those three definitions for PJK that have been used recently (Figure 2):

1. Proximal Junctional angle (PJA) ≥10° and at least 10° more than pre-implantation, with PJA defined as the angle between the caudal endplate of the upper instrumented level to the cephalad endplate 2 vertebrae above the upper instrumented level [21].
2. Proximal Junctional angle (PJA) >10° and at least 10° more than pre-implantation, with PJA defined as the angle between the caudal endplate of 2 vertebrae below the upper instrumented level to the cephalad endplate 2 vertebrae the above upper instrumented level [41].
3. Proximal Junctional angle (PJA) >20°, with PJA defined as the angle between the caudal endplate of the upper instrumented level to the cephalad endplate one vertebrae above the upper instrumented level [42,44].

By employing all three definitions for the same sample of patients, it can be determined if the differences in observed risk were related to the definitions used or the sample of patients that were chosen in each study [43].

El-Hawary et al. [43] conducted an analysis of a group of 36 children with EOS from a multicentre registry who were treated with distraction based systems between 2004 and 2008 with a minimum follow up of two years. His main goal was to determine if different PJK definitions will affect the risk of PJK in the same sample of children, and secondarily to evaluate the reliability of these three different definitions of radiographic PJK. Five observers independently assessed the radiographs for PJK using all three definitions on two separate occasions at least two weeks apart. Risk of PJK varied between 6% and 39% depending upon the definition that was used. Highest risk was observed with Definition 2 (39%), modest using Definition 1 (22%) and the lowest risk with Definition 3 (6%). The variation found in PJK risk with different definitions used was similar to what was observed in the 2011 studies (i.e., Definition 2 yielded the highest risk and Definition 3 yielded the lowest risk).

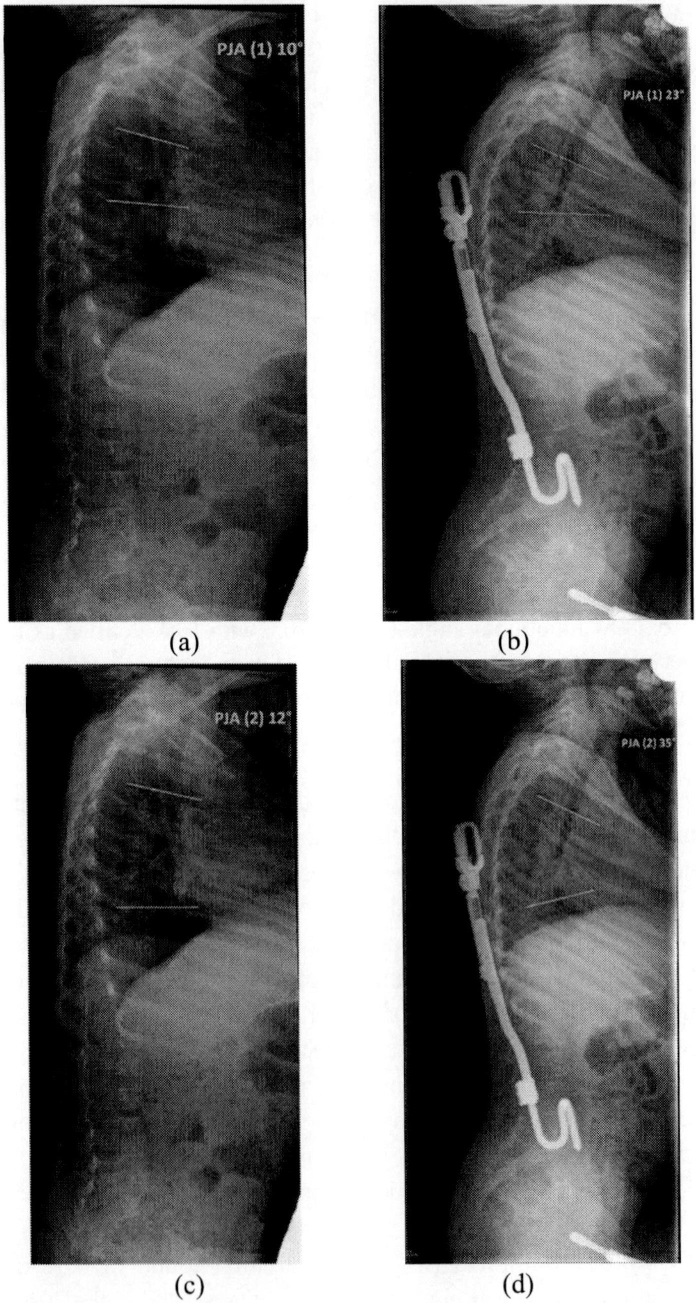

Figure 2. (Continued).

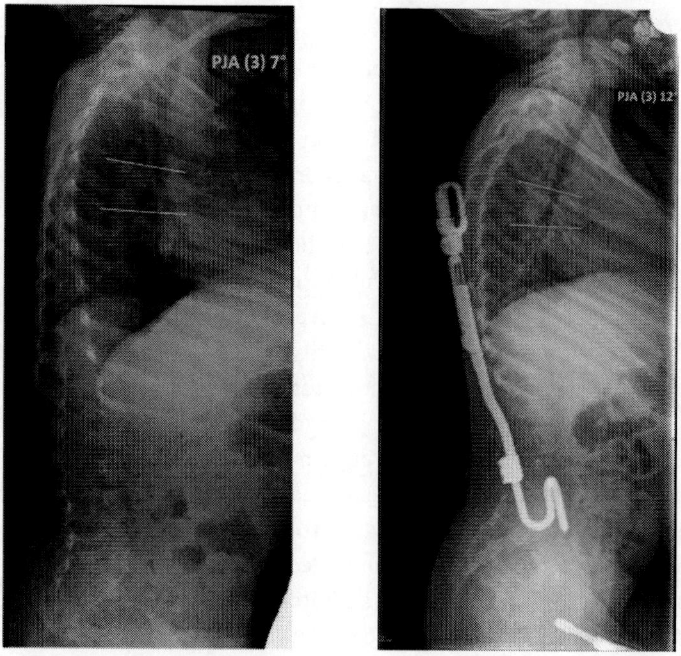

(e) (f)

Figure 2. Eight-year old female patient with Early Onset Scoliosis who was treated with a single Rib-Pelvis construct at the age of three years. Two years post-operatively, she developed proximal implant migration and radiographic PJK as per definitions 1 and 2. (a, b) Pre-and post-operative radiographs demonstrate radiographic PJK as per definition 1. (c, d) Pre-and post-operative radiographs demonstrate radiographic PJK as per definition 2. (e, f) Pre-and post-operative radiographs do not demonstrate radiographic PJK as per definition 3.

The segment length (number of vertebral levels measured) and the angular threshold (10° vs. 20°) used to define PJK influenced the measured risk of PJK. For instance, by including more levels with lower angular threshold (10°), the resultant risk of developing PJK was high (i.e., Definition 2=39%). In contrast, by including fewer levels with a higher angular threshold (20°), the resultant risk of developing PJK was low (i.e., Definition 3 = 6% risk). The use of a unified definition of PJK should improve the consistency of reporting this complication in future studies. Despite the difficulties of analyzing conventional radiographs taken at different institutions, as well as the presence of anatomical and positional variability, better inter and intra-observer agreement was observed with definition 2 than with the other two definitions.

Li et al. [44] in his case series of 68 patients treated with VEPTR found that PJK developed in 6% as was illustrated earlier. He identified that Patients with preoperative thoracic hyperkyphosis may be at higher risk and that PJK often develops within the first year of VEPTR treatment, and that the presence of weak paraspinal muscular support in neuromuscular patients might also place them at higher risk for PJK. Reinker et al. [45] found that upper cradle placement below the third rib, distal anchor placement at too proximal a level, and recurrent erosion and loss of fixation on the proximal ribs contributed to progression of thoracic kyphosis. Thus, he recommended placing the upper cradle at the second rib, distal extension of the construct to the pelvis, and using bilateral implants. In contrast Li current results demonstrate that bilateral rib-to-pelvis constructs do not necessarily prevent progression of thoracic hyperkyphosis. He identified indications for revision surgery to be a deformity sufficiently severe to endanger the neural elements, or the concern that a further increase in the deformity would necessitate a far more difficult and dangerous revision technique. In his small case series, half of the patients who developed PJK were revised to growing rods. Both of those patients required superior extension of the upper instrumented level to correct the PJK.

El-Hawary et al. [43] identified a similar risk of developing PJK between rib-based (25%) and spine-base distraction (31%). In that multicenter study, risk factors for developing PJK included pre-operative thoracic hyperkyphosis and older age at insertion of implants [43]. The identification of pre-operatively high thoracic kyphosis as a risk factor towards developing post-operative PJK may be related to the evidence that demonstrates that growth friendly treatments that require repetitive posterior lengthening procedures are believed to be kyphogenic by nature [40]. Immediately post -operatively, 20% of the subjects already had radiographic PJK along with increased cervical lordosis, which was likely a compensatory mechanism for the PJK. At final post-operative follow-up, 27.5% of subjects had developed radiographic PJK. This group of patients with PJK at minimum two year follow up had persistently higher cervical lordosis and a higher proximal junctional angle as compared to those subjects that did not develop PJK (Figure 3). This study also identified a potential link between high pelvic incidence and the development of PJK that requires further study [43].

Akbarnia et al. [46] reviewed the literature on the complications of growth friendly surgery in EOS, he came to a conclusion that, to avoid proximal junctional kyphosis, the rods should be contoured into kyphosis at the top of the construct and that the interspinous ligaments should be kept intact as much as possible.

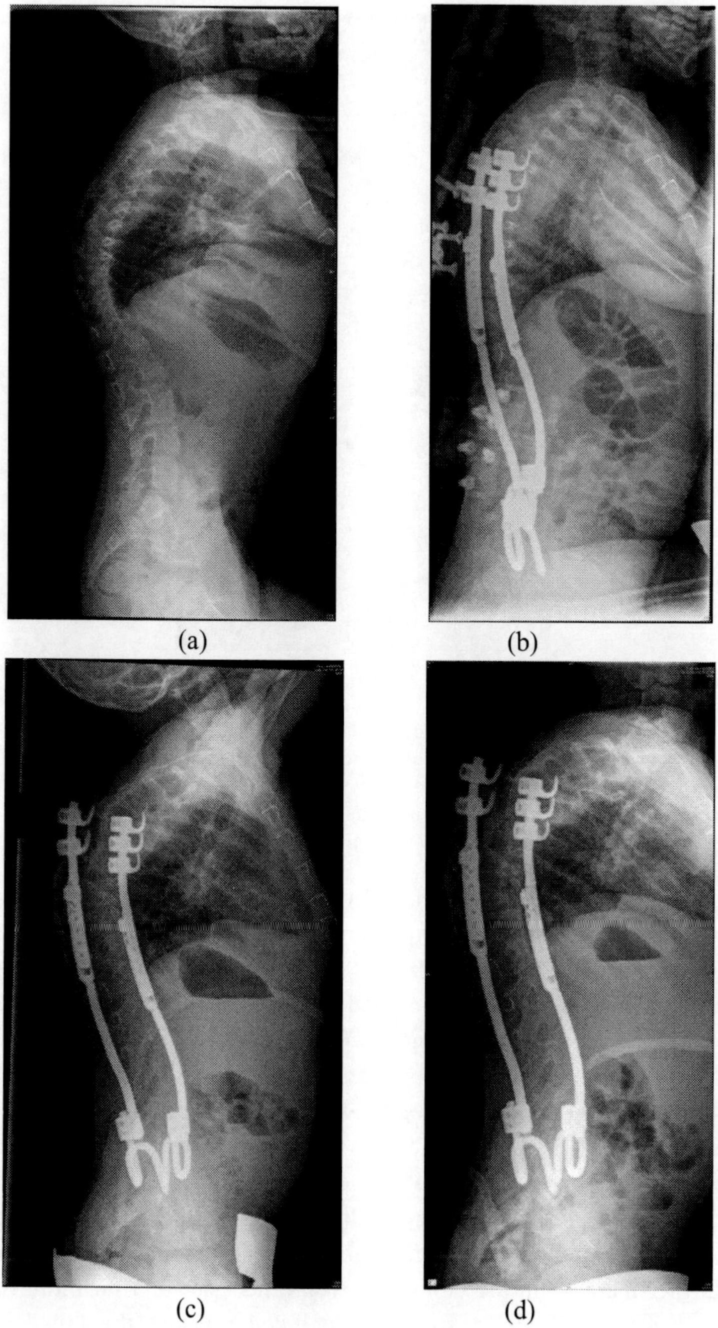

(a) (b) (c) (d)

Figure 3. (Continued).

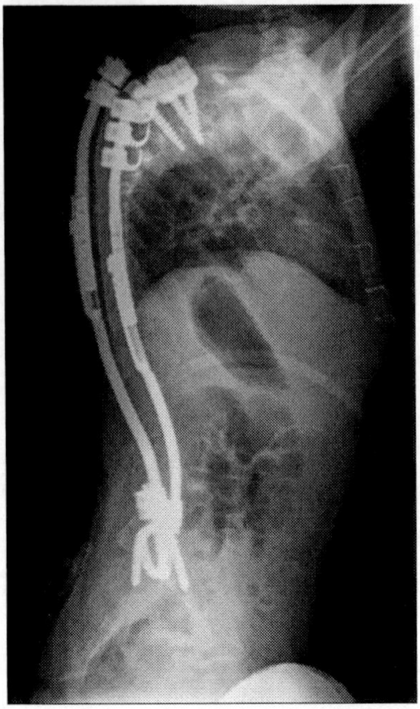

(e)

Figure 3. (a) Pre-operative lateral radiograph of a 4-year old female patient with Early Onset Scoliosis who was treated with two rib-pelvis implants. (b) Immediate post-operative lateral radiograph. (c) Two month post-operative lateral radiograph demonstrates increased cervical lordosis. (d) Six-month post-operative lateral radiograph demonstrates PJK. (e) Lateral radiograph post-revision surgery with proximal extension of implants.

Also extending the upper foundation to at least T2 and avoiding short segment instrumentation might help decrease the risk of PJK. He also believed that excessive upper thoracic kyphosis is a relative contraindication to rib-based distraction and is better handled with spine-based treatment. This is primarily because, unlike first generation rib-based implants, spine-based implants can be continued into the uppermost thoracic or lower cervical spine for control of upper thoracic kyphotic deformity.

Ultimately, PJK is a radiographic parameter. We believe that it may also predispose to implant failure and to the choice of upper instrumented level during revision or graduate surgery. Indications for revision surgery include a deformity sufficiently severe to endanger the neural elements, or the concern that a further increase in the deformity would necessitate a far more difficult revision technique. Revision surgeries included revising the failed implant (rods) to include more cephalad vertebrae, revising rib-based into spine-based rods and definitive fusion techniques. Further studies should be performed to determine what amount of radiographic PJK may be predictive of these clinically relevant complications and the need for surgical intervention.

Conclusion

Proximal junctional kyphosis in early onset scoliosis is a newly recognized complication of growth friendly surgery that may be related to pre-operative thoracic hyperkyphosis as well as to the kyphogenic nature of repetitive posterior distraction surgeries. The risk of developing post-operative PJK in this population ranges from 7% to 56% depending upon the definition used. Utilizing a PJK definition that encompasses more levels measured and a lower angular threshold results in the most reliable measurement of radiographic PJK. The type of implant system, rib-based versus spine-based, does not appear to affect the risk of developing PJK; however, by contouring the rods into kyphosis and by anchoring the rods into the upper thoracic spine, there may be a protective effect on the development of PJK. Links between pre-operative spinopelvic parameters and the development of post-operative PJK requires further study to establish a true relationship. As well, further research is underway to determine how radiographic PJK may ultimately affect clinically relevant patient outcomes.

References

[1] James JI, Lloyd-Roberts GC, Pilcher MF: Infantile structural scoliosis. *J Bone Joint Surg Br* 1959;41:719-735.

[2] Dimeglio A: Growth of the spine before age 5 years. *J Pediatr Orthop B* 1993;1:102-107.

[3] Emery JL, Mithal A: The number of alveoli in the terminal respiratory unit of man during late intrauterine life and childhood. *Arch Dis Child* 1960; 35:544-547.

[4] Williams BA, Matsumoto H, McCalla DJ et al. Development and initial validation of the classification of early-onset scoliosis (C-EOS). *J Bone Joint Surg Am* 2014; 96: 1359-67

[5] Campbell RM Jr, Smith MD, Mayes TC, et al: The characteristics of thoracic insufficiency syndrome associated with fused ribs and congenital scoliosis, *J Bone Joint Surg Am* 85:399, 2003.

[6] James JI, Lloyd-Roberts GC, Pilcher MF: Infantile structural scoliosis. *J Bone Joint Surg Br* 1959;41:719-735.

[7] Mac-Thiong JM, Berthonnaud IE, Dimar JR, et al. Sagittal alignment of the spine and pelvis during growth. *Spine* (Phila Pa 1976) 2004;29:1642e7.

[8] Mac-Thiong JM, Labelle H, Roussouly P, et al. Pediatric sagittal alignment. *Eur Spine J* 2011; 20:S586–S590.

[9] El-Hawary R, Sturm PF, Cahill PJ, Samdani AF, Vitale MG, Gabos PG, Bodin ND, d'Amato CR, Harris C, Howard JJ, Morris SH, Smith JT, et al. Sagittal Spinopelvic Parameters of Young Children With Scoliosis. *Spine Deformity* 1 2013; 343-347.

[10] Goldberg CJ, Gillic I, Connaughton O, et al. Respiratory function and cosmesis at maturity in infantile-onset scoliosis. *Spine* (Phila Pa 1976). 2003;28:2397–2406.

[11] Pehrsson K, Bake B, Larsson S, et al: Lung function in adult idiopathic scoliosis: a 20 year follow up, *Thorax* 46:474, 1991.

[12] Skaggs DL, Akbarnia BA, Flynn JM, Myung KS, Sponseller PD, Vitale MG, et al. A Classification of Growth Friendly Spine Implants. *J Pediatr Orthop* 2013;00:000–000.

[13] Tello CA, et al. Harrington instrumentation without arthrodesis and consecutive distraction program for young children with severe spinal deformities. Experience and technical details. *Orthop Clin North Am.* 1994;25:333–351.

[14] Motoyama EK, Yang CI, Deeney VF, et al. Thoracic malformation with early-onset scoliosis: effect of serial VEPTR expansion thoracoplasty on lung growth and function in children. *Paediatr Respir Rev.* 2009;10:12–17.

[15] Stokes IA, Spence H, Aronsson DD, et al. Mechanical modulation of vertebral body growth. Implications for scoliosis progression. *Spine (Phila Pa 1976).* 1996;21:1162–1167.

[16] Sankar W. N., Acevedo D. C., Skaggs D. L. Comparison of Complications Among Growing Spinal Implants. *Spine* 2010;35:2091–2096.

[17] Bess S, Akbarnia B.A., Thompson G.H., Sponseller P.D., Shah S.A., El Sebaie H, Boachie-Adjei O., Karlin L.I., Canale S., Poe-Kochert C., Skaggs D.L., et al. Complications of Growing-Rod Treatment for Early-

Onset Scoliosis: Analysis of One Hundred and Forty Patients. *J Bone Joint Surg Am.* 2010;92:2533-2543.

[18] Watanabe K., Uno K., Suzuki T., Kawakami N., Tsuji T., Yanagida H, Ito M., Hirano T., Yamazaki K., Minami S., Kotani T., Taneichi H., Imagama S., Takeshita K., Yamamoto T., Matsumoto M., et al. Risk Factors for Complications Associated With Growing-Rod Surgery for Early-Onset Scoliosis. *Spine* 2013;38:E464–E468.

[19] Lucas G, Bollini G, Jouve JL, de Gauzy JS, Accadbled F, Lascombes P, Journeau P, Karger C, Mallet JF, Neagoe P, Cottalorda J, De Billy B, Langlais J,Herbaux B, Fron D, Violas P, et al. Complications in pediatric spine surgery using the vertical expandable prosthetic titanium rib: the French experience. *Spine* (Phila Pa 1976). 2013 Dec 1;38(25):E1589-99.

[20] Schroerlucke S.R., MD, Akbarnia B.A., Pawelek J. B., Salar P., Mundis G.M., Yazici M., Emans J.B., Sponseller P.D., et al., and Growing Spine Study Group*. How Does Thoracic Kyphosis Affect Patient Outcomes in Growing Rod Surgery?. *Spine* 2012; 37 :1303 – 1309.

[21] Glattes RC, Bridwell KH, Lenke LG, Kim YJ, Rinella A, Edwards II C, et al. PJK. Proximal Junctional Kyphosis in Adult Spinal Deformity Following Long Instrumented Posterior Spinal Fusion. Incidence, Outcomes, and Risk Factor Analysis. *Spine* 2005;30:1643–1649.

[22] Kim YJ, Bridwell KH, Lenke LG, Glattes CR, Rhim S, Cheh G, et al. Proximal Junctional Kyphosis in Adult Spinal Deformity After Segmental Posterior Spinal Instrumentation and Fusion. Minimum Five-Year Follow-up. *Spine* 2008;33:2179–2184.

[23] Maruo K, Ha Y, Inoue S, Samuel S, Okada E, Hu SS, Deviren V, Burch S, William S, Ames CP, Mummaneni PV, Chou D, Berven SH, et al. Predictive Factors for Proximal Junctional Kyphosis in Long Fusions to the Sacrum in Adult Spinal Deformity. *Spine* 2013;38:E1469–E1476.

[24] Yagi M, King AB, Boachie-Adjei O et al. Incidence, Risk Factors, and Natural Course of Proximal Junctional Kyphosis. *Surgical Outcomes Review of Adult Idiopathic Scoliosis. Minimum 5 Years of Follow-up. Spine* 2012; 37 : 1479 – 1489.

[25] Yagi M, Akilah KB, Boachie-Adjei O, et al. Incidence, Risk Factors and Classification of Proximal Junctional Kyphosis: Surgical Outcomes Review of Adult Idiopathic Scoliosis.. *Spine* 2010;36:E60–E68.

[26] Kim YJ, Lenke LG, Bridwell KH, Kim J, Cho SK, Cheh G, Yoon J et al. Proximal Junctional Kyphosis in Adolescent Idiopathic Scoliosis After 3 Different Types of Posterior Segmental Spinal Instrumentation

and Fusions Incidence and Risk Factor Analysis of 410 Cases. *Spine* 2007;32:2731–2738.

[27] Lonner BS, Newton P, Betz R, et al. Operative management of Scheuermann's kyphosis in 78 patients: radiographic outcomes, complications, and technique. *Spine (Phila Pa 1976)* 2007; 32:2644 – 52.

[28] Denis F, Sun EC, Winter RB. Incidence and risk factors for proximal and distal junctional kyphosis following surgical treatment for Scheuermann kyphosis: minimum fi ve-year follow-up. *Spine (Phila Pa 1976)* 2009; 34: E729 – 34.

[29] Wang J, Zhao Y, Shen B, et al. Risk factor analysis of proximal junctional kyphosis after posterior fusion in patients with idiopathic scoliosis. *Injury* 2010; 41: 415 – 20.

[30] Kim HJ, Yagi M, Nyugen J, et al. Combined anterior-posterior surgery is the most important risk factor for developing proximal junctional kyphosis in idiopathic scoliosis. *Clin Orthop Relat Res* 2012; 470: 1633 – 9.

[31] Mendoza-Lattes S, Ries Z, Gao Y, et al. Proximal junctional kyphosis in adult reconstructive spine surgery results from incomplete restoration of the lumbar lordosis relative to the magnitude of the thoracic kyphosis. *Iowa Orthop J* 2011; 31: 199 – 206.

[32] Carman DL, Browne RH, Birch JG. Measurement of scoliosis and kyphosis radiographs: intraobserver and interobserver variation. *J Bone Joint Surg* 1990;72-A:328–33.

[33] Kim HJ, Lenke LG, Shaffrey CI, Van Alstyne EM, Skelly AC, et al. Proximal Junctional Kyphosis as a Distinct Form of Adjacent Segment Pathology After Spinal Deformity Surgery. *A Systematic Review. Spine* 2012; 37: S144 – S164.

[34] Hostin R, McCarthy I, O'Brien M, Bess S, Line B, Boachie-Adjei O, Burton D, Gupta M, Ames C, Deviren V, Kebaish K, Shaffrey C, Wood K, Hart R, International Spine Study Group, et al. Incidence, Mode, and Location of Acute Proximal Junctional Failures After Surgical Treatment of Adult Spinal Deformity. *Spine* 2013; 38:1008 – 1015.

[35] Lee GA, Betz RR, Clements DH III, et al. Proximal kyphosis after posterior spinal fusion in patients with idiopathic scoliosis. *Spine* 1999;24:795–9.

[36] Helgeson M. D., Shah S. A., Newton P. O., et al. Evaluation of proximal junctional kyphosis in adolescent idiopathic scoliosis following pedicle

screw, hook, or hybrid instrumentation. *Spine* (Phila Pa 1976). 2010; 35(2): 177-81.

[37] Yang S. H., Chen P. Q. Proximal kyphosis after short posterior fusion for thoracolumbar scoliosis. Clin Orthop Relat Res. 2003; 411): 152-8.

[38] Rhee J. M., Bridwell K. H., Won D. S., et al. Sagittal plane analysis of adolescent idiopathic scoliosis: the effect of anterior versus posterior instrumentation. *Spine* (Phila Pa 1976). 2002; 27(21): 2350-6.

[39] Kang M. M., Bridwell K. H., Lenke L. G., et al. Proximal Junctional Kyphosis in Primary Adult Deformity Surgery: Evaluation of 20 Degrees as a Critical Angle. *Neurosurgery.* 2013.

[40] El-Hawary R., Sturm P., Cahill P., et al. Sagittal Spinopelvic Parameters Help Predict the Risk of Proximal Junctional Kyphosis for Children Treated with Posterior Distraction Based Implants. The 5th International Congress on Early Onset Scoliosis and Growing Spine (ICEOS); Orlando, Florida. *Journal of Children's Orthopaedics Springer-Verlag;* 2011. p. 387-401.

[41] Skaggs D., Myung K., Lee C. Proximal Junctional Kyphosis in Distraction-Based Growing Rods. The 5th International Congress on Early Onset Scoliosis and Growing Spine (ICEOS); Orlando, Florida. Journal of Children's Orthopaedics: Springer-Verlag; 2011. p. 387-401.

[42] Li Y., Karlin L. Proximal Segmental Kyphosis After Vertical Expandable Prosthetic Titanium Rib Insertion. The 5th International Congress on Early Onset Scoliosis and Growing Spine (ICEOS); Orlando, Florida. *Journal of Children's Orthopaedics:* Springer-Verlag; 2011. p. 387-401.

[43] El-Hawary R., Al Khudairy A., Gauthier L., Heflin J., Fletcher N., Matz J., Sorocean A., et al. Reliability of Proximal Junctional Kyphosis Measurements for Young Children With Scoliosis. Spine Deformity 2 (2014) 448-453.

[44] Li Y., Meryl G., Karlin L. Proximal Junctional Kyphosis After Vertical Expandable Prosthetic Titanium Rib Insertion. *Spine Deformity* 2013; 1 (6): 425-33.

[45] Reinker K, Simmons JW, Patil V, et al. Can VEPTR control progression of early-onset kyphoscoliosis? A cohort study of VEPTR patients with severe kyphoscoliosis. *Clin Orthop Relat Res* 2011;469:1342e8.

[46] Akbarnia B.A., Emans J. B. Complications of Growth-Sparing Surgery in Early Onset Scoliosis. *Spine* 2010;35:2193–2204.

In: Kyphosis
Editor: Janice Newton

ISBN: 978-1-63483-224-3

Chapter III

Cervical Kyphotic Deformity Evaluation and Management

Stephen K. Huo, Young Lu, Martin Eichler and S. Samuel Bederman
University of California, Irvine, Medical Center, Department of Orthopaedic Surgery, Pavillion III, Orange, CA, US

Abstract

Kyphosis is the most common spinal deformity of the cervical spine. Patients may present with progressive deformity and adverse associated consequences, including neck pain, neurologic dysfunction, postural instability, and a marked decline in health-related quality of life. As patients develop further progression of kyphosis, neck pain, inability to achieve horizontal gaze, and neurological deficits may worsen due to a combination of nerve root or spinal cord traction. In this circumstance, surgical correction of kyphosis has been shown to have the most pivotal role in improving clinical results.

Although many patients with cervical kyphosis (CK) present with similar complaints, numerous etiologies have been reported, including trauma, neoplasm, post-radiation, degenerative disease, systemic arthritides, neuromuscular disorders, infection, and iatrogenic conditions (e.g., following cervical laminectomy). Determining the specific cause is critical to appreciate the unique precautions and considerations that may influence the approach to treatment. A thorough, systematic clinical and radiographic evaluation of every patient is necessary to direct appropriate treatment, both non-operative and surgical.

For relatively mild cases of cervical deformity without neurologic deficits, non-operative treatment with activity modification, physical therapy, or bracing can be considered. However, for severe, progressively worsening deformity with evidence of neurologic deficits, or chin-on-chest deformity affecting the ability to achieve horizontal gaze, surgical intervention is recommended. Although surgery may be performed by anterior, posterior, or combined approaches, the decision on which approach and, if necessary, a particular sequence of staged approaches is based on both patient-specific factors and surgeon preference. In general, kyphosis correction is obtained by lengthening the anterior column of the spine, shortening the posterior column of the spine, or a combination of both. Because of the proximity of the spinal cord, nerve roots, and vertebral arteries, it may be necessary to correct in multiple stages with several approaches. Many combinations of the above approaches have been described in the literature, each with their respective advantages and disadvantages, thus highlighting their differential utility given the patients' presenting condition.

Due to the potentially extensive, prolonged nature of the surgical procedures, surgeons must be cognizant and anticipate for potential post-operative adjuncts to facilitate recovery and reduce complications, such as delayed extubation and consideration of placement of a feeding tube. Furthermore, anticipating potential complications and taking specific precautionary measures with careful pre-operative planning can help reduce the incidence of adverse events post-operatively.

The treatment of patients with cervical kyphosis is challenging. Proper evaluation requires an appreciation of the various causes contributing to the deformity, a thorough understanding of the anatomical structures, and an appreciation of the surgical options available including the use of combined surgical approaches or complex correctional techniques to achieve optimal patient outcomes.

Introduction

Neck pain is the fourth leading cause of disability in the United States with an annual prevalence of 23.1%. Estimated one year incidence of neck pain varies in the literature from 10.4% to 21.3% with most cases occurring in females and office/computer workers [1]. While the majority of cases of neck pain (33-65%) are considered acute and may resolve without treatment, nearly half of patients with neck pain will continue to experience recurrent episodes of pain and discomfort [2]. The incidence of cervical degenerative myelopathy or radiculopathy, however, is significantly lower with a point prevalence of 3.5 per 1,000 popuation3 and an annual incidence of 0.83 per 1,000 population [3, 4]. While the actual overall incidence of cervical kyphotic (CK) deformity is unknown due to its multifactorial etiologies (trauma, neoplasm, post-radiation, degenerative disease, systemic arthritides, neuromuscular disorders, infection, and iatrogenic conditions), it is likely that only a small proportion of neck pain is due to kyphotic deformity of the cervical spine. Le Huec et al. reported a kyphotic subaxial cervical spine in one third of an asymptomatic population (ODI < 20% and VAS < 2), indicating that the physiological cervical lordosis is not always favorable in an energetic balanced spine [5].

Although cervical kyphosis only represents a small percentage of patients with neck pain, the presence of this deformity can greatly diminish a patient's quality of life. Several authors have established a clear relationship between global and regional sagittal alignment parameters (sagittal vertical alignment) and clinical outcomes [6-8]. Cervical kyphosis leading to chin-on-chest deformity can result in difficulty in maintaining horizontal gaze, which can severely impair a patient's ability to ambulate. Furthermore, neutral cervical alignment requires intact function of the posterior cervical musculature to maintain acceptable head posture. The subsequent fatiguing of the cervical musculature can, in addition to kyphotic deformity, also lead to constant unremitting pain and discomfort. The need to maintain an acceptable horizontal gaze can also result in a compensatory lumbar hyperlordosis, thus, in turn, leading to low back pain [9]. Severe cases of cervical kyphosis can also lead to cervical myelopathy or induce progression of existing myelopathy [9]. This relationship is supported by a cadaveric study and a retrospective imaging study demonstrating that progressive kyphosis of the cervical spine reduces spinal canal dimensions and increases spinal cord intramedullary pressure [10, 11]. In more severe cases, this deformity can also lead to dysphagia or even respiratory difficulties [9]. In addition to neck pain, deformity, and neurological dysfunction, the presence of cervical kyphosis may even lead to progression of kyphosis. The normal sagittal weight-bearing axis lies posterior to the cervical vertebral bodies, and therefore about two thirds of the forces are transmitted through the posterior elements [12]. The advantage of this anatomic relationship is that it maintains cervical sagittal balance while also reducing the mechanical demand on the posterior musculature of the cervical spine. As the cervical spine undergoes kyphotic collapse, however, the weight-bearing axis is shifted anteriorly, thereby placing increased forces on the anterior elements and also placing the posterior cervical musculature at a mechanical disadvantage. In turn, as the posterior musculature fatigues and the anterior elements collapse due to the abnormally increased axial load, further kyphotic collapse results [9, 12].

Surgical strategies for treating cervical kyphosis should be aimed at correcting and stabilizing the deformity, achieving sagittal balance, and decompressing neural elements. Proper pre-operative planning utilizing various cervico-occipital parameters to assess the sagittal balance is essential. The choice of surgical approach is generally dependent on the relative flexibility of the dorsal versus ventral aspects of the cervical spine. Once the surgical approach is determined, correction of flexible kyphosis can be attained with simple reduction and instrumentation, whereas rigid kyphosis may require additional osteotomies followed by instrumentation and fusion.

Etiologies of Cervical Kyphosis

The most well studied etiology of cervical kyphosis is an iatrogenic process arising most commonly following cervical laminectomy. However, any pathology that induces instability or collapse of the anterior or posterior columns of the cervical spine can produce a gradual loss of sagittal spinal balance, thereby promoting kyphosis of the cervical spine. Cervical kyphosis can occur following any degenerative disease, trauma, neoplasia, radiation therapy, infection, or systemic conditions such as ankylosing spondylitis or rheumatoid arthritis, as well as neuromuscular disorders and myopathies.

The most common cause of iatrogenic cervical kyphosis is following prior surgery. Specifically, pseudoarthrosis, failure to restore the desired cervical alignment, or approach-related destabilization could lead to cervical kyphosis. The most common postsurgical deformity is post-laminectomy kyphosis. Destabilization of these posterior structures shifts the weight-bearing axis anteriorly. As the axial load on the anterior elements increases, the anterior column may undergo collapse and wedge deformation leading to cervical kyphosis [12, 13]. The incidence of post-laminectomy kyphosis has been estimated to be as high as 21% in one case series of 42 patients and is highly dependent on the patient's age, preoperative lordosis as well as the extent of laminectomy [13-16]. In general, pediatric and young adults are more likely to develop post-laminectomy kyphosis due to greater laxity of the interspinous ligaments, more horizontal orientation of the facets and incompletely ossified vertebral bodies that are more likely to collapse into kyphosis [17, 18].

Reduced preoperative lordosis can be further aggravated by laminectomies that involve greater number of levels that will generally further destabilize the spine, thereby raising the risk of kyphotic development [9].

Generally, traumatic injury to the posterior ligaments can destabilize the cervical sagittal alignment resulting in a gradual kyphotic collapse. Injuries to the anterior column, such as compression fractures, can produce anterior wedging of the cervical vertebral bodies, which can lead to a kyphotic alignment. In similar fashion, degenerative loss of intervertebral disc space can also result in gradual anterior collapse of the cervical spine [9].

The presence of a tumor, especially a spinal cord tumor involving the anterior horn cells, can result in denervation and weakness of the posterior cervical musculature. This loss of posterior muscle tone can also be a contributing cause or accelerate cervical kyphotic deformity. An important example of a neoplasia-associated cervical kyphosis is neurofibromatosis type I (NF-1). Although cervical kyphosis arising from NF-1 is relatively rare, spinal manifestations are the most common orthopedic manifestation of NF-1 [19]. The pathophysiology of NF-1 associated kyphosis is unknown but is likely due to endocrine abnormalities, mesodermal dysplasia, or the mass effect of tumors localized in the cervical spine. An important aspect in the management of NF-1 related cervical kyphosis is that the deformity is associated with key morphologic changes including spindling of the transverse processes, erosive changes involving the posterior margins of the vertebral bodies, and enlarged neural foramina, all of which may increase the technical complexities of surgical correction. Moreover, dysmorphic pedicle dimensions, which are commonly seen in NF1-related cervical kyphosis, may prevent the use of pedicle screws, thereby necessitating the use of alternative fixation techniques, such as lateral mass screws. Lastly, the presence of the lesion may also lead to intraoperative hemorrhage and therefore a pre-operative tumor embolization should be considered [20-24]. Systemic inflammatory arthritides can induce deformity of the cervical spine through weakening of the posterior elements. Ankylosing spondylitis (AS) is a debilitating inflammatory condition that is characterized by an immune-mediated erosion of the axial skeleton and spine. Progressive erosion of the vertebral joints and intervertebral disc spaces along with ossification and auto-fusion can produce severe cervical flexion deformities. Due to the severe rigid deformity, patients with AS-mediated cervical kyphosis may have respiratory difficulties that can pose a significant morbidity risk with anesthesia, especially with surgical approaches requiring prone positioning. Dysphagia due to severe cervical kyphosis in AS can lead to nutritional deficiencies, which can affect postoperative recovery and healing. In turn, both the pulmonary and swallowing functions of these patients need to be properly addressed prior to surgery [25-30].

Similar to inflammatory arthritides, infections of the cervical spine that erode the anterior body and weaken the posterior columns can also produce cervical kyphosis. While disseminated tuberculosis generally affects the thoracic or lumbar spine, it is theoretically possible for mycobacteria to infect the cervical vertebral bodies. Tuberculosis generally has a predilection for the anterior aspects of the vertebral body and has a tendency to affect children more than adults. [31]. In children, disseminated tuberculosis generally results in buckling collapse with complete destruction of the vertebral bodies along with facet dislocation [31]. This pattern of collapse often leads to severe kyphosis and increased risk of subluxation and dislocations, thereby also raising the risk of spinal cord compression and injury [31]. Due to the possibility of pan-vertebral involvement of the spine in tuberculosis-related cervical kyphosis, a pre-operative MRI is recommended to assess the pathologic involvement of the pedicles, vertebral body and disc, and the presence of prevertebral abscesses [32].

Abnormal and asymmetric tone of the cervical spine musculature can lead to a so-called 'dropped head syndrome'. It is either caused by excessive tension of the anterior or declined strength of the posterior cervical muscle. The former is associated with multiple system atrophy, whereas the latter includes amyotrophic lateral sclerosis, myasthenia gravis, and polymyositis. [33]. Other associated diseases such as multiple sclerosis, polymyositis, Charcot-Marie-Tooth disease as well as extrapyramidal disorders such as Parkinson's disease, can also produce gradual anterior collapse of cervical sagittal alignment.

Treatment with anti-Parkinsonian drugs can alleviate symptoms in some patients but may trigger or aggravate the condition in others. Case series by Kashihara et al. demonstrated that the onset of cervical kyphosis in Parkinsonian patients following initiation of a dopamine agonist was alleviated with changes in the anti-Parkinsonian medication regimen [34]. Idiopathic Senile CK is a diagnosis of exclusion in patient presenting with dropped head syndrome. Neuromuscular diseases should be excluded with a thorough neurological examination including electrophysiological examination, MRI of the head and cervical spine and biopsy of the extensor neck muscles. The latter will show non-specific myopathic features without inflammation [33]. Blood analysis could detect endocrinological diseases such as hypothyroidism and diabetes as well as Myasthenia gravis, which is identified by a Tensilon test.

Since the overall prognosis is favorable, an individual muscle strength program is advised [35]. Surgical intervention should be considered if neurological symptoms due to myelopathy or radiculopathy are present.

Overall, kyphotic deformity of the cervical spine is a debilitating condition that can arise following any pathology that weakens the posterior elements and abnormally loads the weight-bearing axis anteriorly. For adequately addressing cervical kyphosis, careful consideration to the underlying etiology must be taken in regards to surgical planning.

Assessment

A complete clinical evaluation of the patient, composed of a thorough history, physical examination, and relevant imaging, is a crucial step for assessing cervical kyphotic deformities and for determining the most appropriate patient-specific treatment [25]. While the clinical presentation may be similar across patients with cervical kyphosis, the surgeon must attempt to recognize the various contributing etiologies, as certain conditions may require unique precautions influencing the treatment approach [36].

Common complaints elicited from patients include neck pain/stiffness, progressive neurologic symptoms, and worsening deformity causing functional impairments, such as difficulty maintaining horizontal gaze or dysphagia [37]. Patients with severe fixed deformities may also present with lower back pain attributable to positional compensations to maintain overall sagittal balance. Pertinent details, such as ongoing use of nonsteroidal anti-inflammatory drugs for concern of pseudoarthrosis, smoking history, prior history of cervical trauma or surgeries, baseline nutritional assessment from difficulties swallowing, and relevant causative co-morbidities, should be elicited for consideration when tailoring treatment options.

The patient should be evaluated standing upright, laying supine, and in the sitting position, as each of these physical examination components provide various pieces of information regarding the nature of the deformity and help identify the primary location of deformity. While standing with the knees and hips completely extended and maintaining the neck in a neutral position, the Chin-Brow Vertical Angle (CBVA) can be estimated using a line connecting the chin to brow and the angle subtended by a vertical line tangent to the floor (Figure 1). Although the definitive normal value for CBVA has not been determined, a spinal correction ranging from +10 to -10 degrees has been shown to be generally well tolerated. The significance of the CBVA is that it can provide an estimate of the size of the posterior osteotomy wedge needed to restore extension in fixed variants [38, 39]. Overall, use of the CBVA has been gaining favor, as correction of the CBVA has been correlated with improved post-operative patient outcomes, such as ambulation, horizontal gaze, and in conducting activities of daily living [12, 25]. While laying flat, the stiffness of the deformity can be evaluated, as patients with rigid deformities will present with cervical flexion that persists even while in the supine position, whereas patients with deformities elsewhere (e.g., lumbar flatback, thoracic hyperkyphosis, or hip deformities) will compensate or correct. The sitting position eliminates contributing effects of any potential lumbar and hip/pelvis deformities [25, 40].

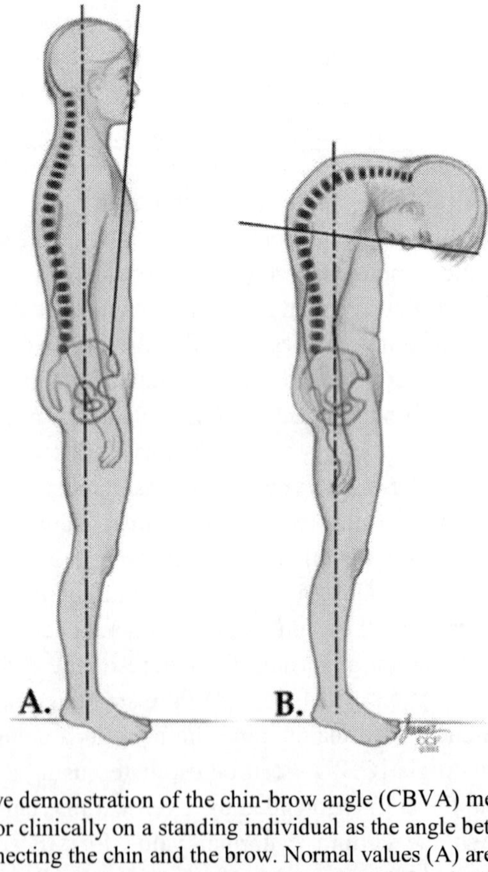

Figure 1. Illustrative demonstration of the chin-brow angle (CBVA) measured on either a lateral radiograph or clinically on a standing individual as the angle between a vertical axis line and a line connecting the chin and the brow. Normal values (A) are close to 0 degrees, which is in stark comparison to patients with chin-on-chest deformity (B). (Reprinted with permission. Cleveland Clinic Center Photography © 2011-2012. All rights reserved).

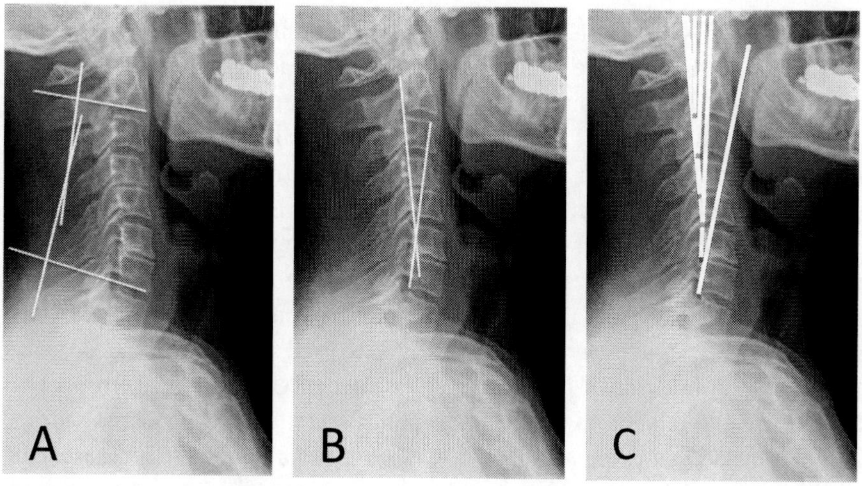

Figure 2. The 3 radiographic sagittal assessment of cervical alignment includes the Cobb Angle (A), Jackson physiological stress line (B), and the Harrison posterior tangent method (C).

Radiographic evaluation for all patients is comprised of anteroposterior (AP), lateral cervical plain radiographs, and dynamic lateral flexion/extension views to help evaluate for the flexibility of the cervical region and to rule out atlanto-axial instability especially in rheumatoid disease. In addition, a full length standing 36-inch lateral and posteroanterior (PA) view is useful for assessing global spinal balance [25].

From the lateral cervical radiograph, the three primary radiographic methods to assess cervical alignment can be obtained. These measures include the Cobb angle, the Harrison posterior tangent method, and the Jackson physiological stress lines (Figure 2) [41]. The Cobb angle method is arguably the most commonplace clinical method of evaluating cervical lordosis and can best be measured from C2 to C7. Calculating the Cobb angle utilizes a line drawn parallel to the inferior endplate of C2 or from a line connecting the C1 anterior tubercle to the spinous process and, in similar fashion, a second line is drawn parallel to the C7 inferior endplate, after which lines perpendicular to both the aforementioned lines are drawn, the subsequent angle created from the intersecting lines provides the Cobb angle. The Jackson physiological stress line method involves a line parallel to the posterior aspect of the C2 and C7 vertebral body and measuring the angle created by the intersecting lines [12]. The Harrison posterior tangent method is comprised of drawing lines parallel to the posterior aspect of the C2 to C7 vertebral bodies, then summating the subsequent supplemental angles to obtain the angle of overall curvature [12, 41]. Despite concerns of inaccurate readings from Cobb method depending on the proximal extent of the measurement, the Cobb method remains the most widely utilized method for analyzing cervical lordosis, presumably in part due to its high inter-rater and intra-rater reliability and its straightforward application [12, 42, 43].

The conventional CBVA, which assesses the extent of horizontal gaze clinically, can also be measured radiographically from the lateral view of a standing 36-inch plain film. For gauging sagittal translational cervical alignment, the sagittal vertical axis (SVA) is used to measure the distance from a plumb line drawn from either the center of C2 or the posterosuperior aspect of C7 in relation to the posterosuperior sacral corner, which provides a global translational assessment [12]. A more regionally defined measurement can be obtained by measuring the distance between the C2 and C7 plumb lines. However, the C2 plumb line method is the more clinically meaningful measurement, as larger values of C2 SVA has been correlated with lower health-related quality of life (Figure 3). C2-C7 SVA values less than 40 mm show significantly better outcomes [7].

More recent studies have concentrated on sagittal balance and have introduced new parameters. Lee et al. postulated that an energetic balanced cervical spine is correlated to the thoracic inlet angle (TIA), an individual constant parameter comparable to the pelvic incidence, that drives the neck tilt (NT) and the T1 slope [44].

The following equation describes the relation between the aforementioned parameters: TIA = T1 slope + NT (Figure 4) [44]. To maintain a physiological neck tilt of 45° and therefore minimize the energy expenditure of the posterior neck musculature, a large thoracic inlet decreases the T1 slope, which drives the cervical subaxial lordosis.

As the amount of neck tilt and the T1 slope are position-dependent and sum to the TIA, which is fixed, as one leans forward, thus decreasing the neck tilt, the T1 slope increases to result in more cervical lordosis. Similarly, as one actively leans backward, thus increasing the neck tilt, the T1 slope decreases resulting in less cervical lordosis. In addition to TIA, other measures have been used to evaluate sagittal balance [5]. Having a proper appreciation of normal cervical sagittal spinal balance, allows us to better predict physiologic alignment and guide deformity correction.

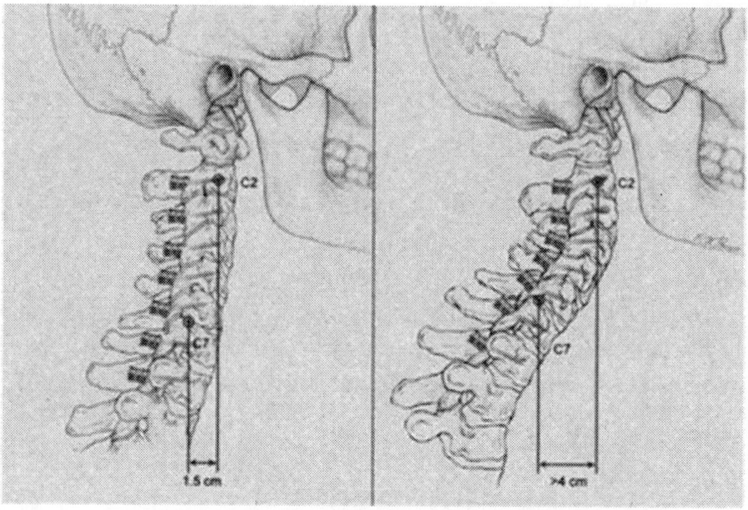

Figure 3. Depiction of the C2 and C7 plumb lines and their respective distances for both a normal cervical spine (A) and a spine with significant cervical kyphotic deformity (B), which illustrates the increasing distance between the two plumb lines with progressive deformity. (From Scheer JK, et al. Cervical spine alignment, sagittal deformity, and clinical implications. Neurosurg Spine 19:141–159, 2013 ©AANS, 2013, with permission).

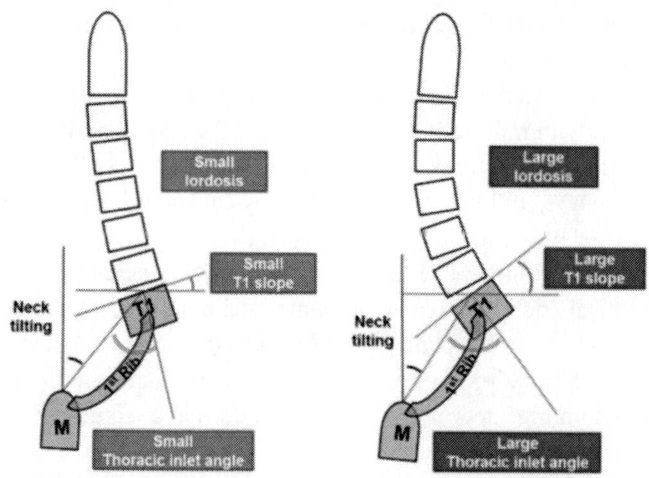

Figure 4. A small thoracic inlet angle yields a low T-1 slope and therefore less cervical lordosis is required to balance the head over the thoracic inlet and trunk. Conversely, a large thoracic inlet angle yields a greater T-1 slope so that a greater magnitude of cervical lordosis is required to balance the head over the thoracic inlet and trunk. M = manubrium. (Reproduced with permission from Lee et al.: *J Spinal Disord Tech 25:*E41–E47, 2012).

Further imaging modalities, such as magnetic resonance imaging (MRI) and computed tomography (CT) scans, can be useful adjuncts for pre-operative planning. MRI is used to assess for spinal cord or nerve root impingement, disc integrity, which may influence the sequence of staged surgeries if decompression is deemed necessary prior to the deformity correction. CT scans can better visualize the osseous structures to plan instrumentation and to assess for the presence of ankylosis in the facet joints or collapse of discs, which will affect the surgical decision-making process. Finally, radiographic details, such as pre-existing surgical changes, aberrant anatomic variants, the presence of pseudoarthrosis or subluxations, should be noted for consideration as part of the pre-operative planning.

Management

Several non-operative regimens directed at alleviating symptoms are available to patients prior to undertaking operative treatment. These conservative measures include use of nonsteroidal anti-inflammatory medications, muscle relaxants, physical therapy for isometric neck musculature strengthening, chiropractic care, bracing or collar trials, and cervical traction [12, 45].

Patients with ankylosing spondylitis as well as those with symptomatic arthropathy but with mild radiographic deformities may benefit from a trial of daily positional modifications to minimize undue neck flexion (such as sleeping without a pillow), bracing therapy or other external stabilizing modalities to delay deformity progression [25]. Patients who have sustained any fractures require urgent clinical and radiographic assessment and should undergo surgical stabilization with some attempt at kyphosis correction. Surgical correction of kyphotic deformities should be considered when patients have exhausted non-operative management, demonstrate severe neck pain or deteriorating neurologic deficits, and have significant deformity leading to functional disabilities, such as loss of horizontal gaze (chin-on-chest deformity) [12, 24]. Specific patient characteristics, such as the underlying etiology, prior surgical histories, and the severity of the deformity should be assessed during the pre-operative phase in order to tailor the most appropriate treatment plan [36]. Generally, larger magnitude deformities are inherently associated with a greater risk of contracting chronic pain post-operatively or neurologic deficits [7]. However, regardless of the various patient-specific factors, the primary objective with surgery is to restore cervical alignment in the sagittal plane so as to improve pain, achieve horizontal gaze, and decompress the neural elements.

The distinction of classifying cervical kyphosis as a fixed or flexible deformity is a crucial initial step in pre-operative planning, as it will dictate the type of surgical approach and intra-operative procedures that are appropriate [46]. Flexible deformities are able to be reduced either by postural positioning or by application of gentle traction, and thus, may be amenable to reduction from a single approach [46]. Fixed deformities, on the other hand, may be more likely to require combined approaches and osteotomies. In the case of a flexible deformity, a single anterior or posterior approach has both been proposed [47-49]. If a single approach can adequately addresses the pathology directly, anteriorly or posteriorly, the associated morbidity can be significantly reduced as compared to an otherwise more extensive combined approach [9, 49].

The overall principle for addressing the cervical kyphotic deformities involve restoring cervical lordosis by either lengthening the anterior column through large interbody or corpectomy grafts or cages, shortening the posterior column with facetectomies or osteotomies, or the combination of both. Although no universal rule regarding the optimal amount of surgical correction/restoration of cervical lordosis exists, most surgeons will generally strive to achieve as close to neutral alignment as possible [45].

During surgical planning, the amount of correction needed and the location of the apex of the deformity should be determined based on appropriate imaging studies, as it will determine the type of osteotomy, number of instrumented levels and type of hardware needed, and potentially the sequence of surgical approaches [45, 50]. However, care should be taken not to overcorrect the deformity, especially in the setting of concomitant lumbar deformity requiring surgical intervention, as this may leave the patient with an upward gaze and unable to visualize the ground in front of them after lumbar correction, precluding the patient from independent ambulation and working at a desk [25, 37]. Generally, lumbar and thoracic sagittal imbalance has to be addressed first prior to correction of the cervical spine (Figure 5).

Although no definitive rule regarding the "correct" amount of post-operative cervical lordotic restoration exists, the general consensus is to restore cervical kyphosis to as close to neutral as possible to allow for horizontal gaze [45]. Radiographic measures, such as TIA may be promising to help in the preoperative planning of the correction.

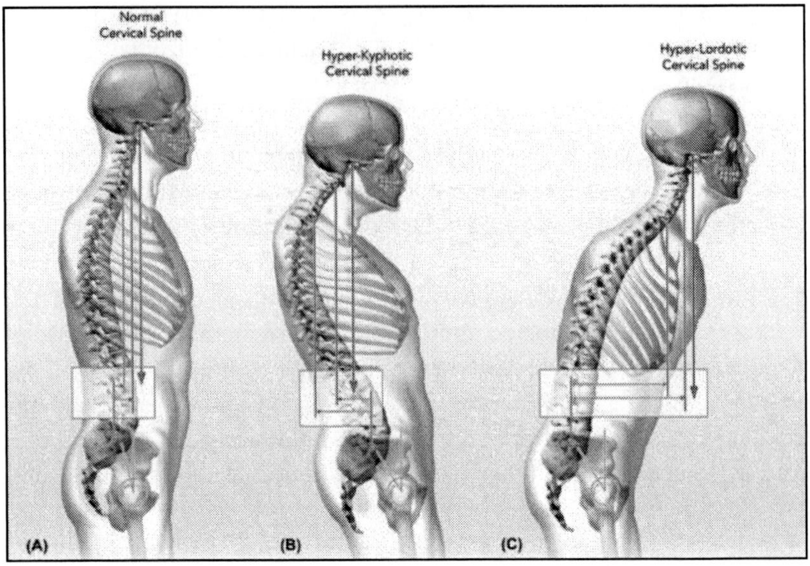

Figure 5. Appropriate sagittal alignment is required for posture maintenance (A) as malalignment leads to compensatory mechanisms (B and C). (Reproduced with permission from Ames et al.: *Spine (Phil Pa 1976)* 38:S149–S160, 2013) [51].

Determining the number of spinal levels to be surgically addressed is a multifactorial decision that is tailored to each patient and their respective circumstances. Variables that need to be considered include the surgical approach, underlying etiology, global versus focal deformity and the deformity profile. Obtaining an adequate deformity correction through a single level at the apex may be challenging, if not impossible, so a more controlled and powerful correction is undertaken by restoring a few degrees of reduction across multiple levels. The summation of the corrections can lead to tremendous improvements in alignment [46].

Some authors advocate for operating only the most caudal and rostral vertebral levels contributing to the deformity curve. However, as adjacent level pathology, such as symptomatic spondylosis or degenerative disease, often accompanies deformities to create a compensatory lordosis in attempts to restore the overall alignment, extension of the fixation length to involve 1-2 "normal" vertebrae may be necessary. A longer construct will also provide a longer moment arm that may be needed to correct and maintain deformities of a larger magnitude [49, 52].

Although the cervical spine can be approached anteriorly or posteriorly for cervical deformity correction, a combination of approaches is often necessary to address the more severe variants. The decision to undertake a single versus multiple approaches, and determining the specific sequence of corrective procedures is a complex process, as the potential advantages and disadvantages of each combination of approach must be considered in addition to the characteristics of the deformity and the patient profile. A single anterior approach should be considered for addressing flexible cervical kyphosis without dorsal pathology, namely facet joint ankylosis [46-48]. The reduction is achieved by distracting the anterior column across implants, interbody fusion can be supplemented for the purpose of anterior column load sharing but is not required for correction of the deformity itself [46-48]. Significantly more surgical leverage can be obtained anteriorly compared to posterior approaches for deformity correction [52]. By utilizing multiple points of fixation, the surgeon can restore cervical lordosis and also perform an anterior decompression. It is usually an effective approach for addressing flexible postsurgical cervical kyphosis.

A one-stage anterior approach has been described for patients with deformities attributed to tuberculosis with good clinical outcomes, which was accompanied with debridement, post-operative chemotherapy, and nutritional supplementation [53]. By utilizing a single approach, patients had minimal complication rates, reduced blood loss, while still attaining adequate kyphotic correction. Advantages also include the relative ease of performing neural decompression as compared to a posterior approach, allowing correction of the deformity from the same surgical approach, and the straightforward instrumentation process. The amount of lordosis restoration that can be achieved at the cervical and cervicothoracic junction is also significantly more than the attainable correction for lumbar and thoracolumbar kyphotic variants [53].

However, surgeons should keep in mind that the amount of correction achieved through a single approach will be relatively limited and may have a higher non-union rate compared to a combined approach. Also, if the region of the cervical spine necessitating corpectomies for corrective purposes spans equal or greater than three levels or if the bone quality is deemed poor, a supplemental posterior fusion and instrumentation is recommended [9, 49, 54].

A single posterior approach may be useful for flexible deformities that reduce completely upon extension or with traction and in the absence of significant anterior ankylosis [9]. For mild, flexible degenerative kyphotic deformities, the use of cervical pedicle screw fixation to correct the deformity has been described [55]. However, its applicable utility is limited given the risks of pedicle screw placement across the entire cervical spine. Although the prospect of alternative fixation, such as lateral mass screws, can be considered, due to their inherently weaker fixation, we cannot recommend a suboptimal construct for the sake of a single approach, even for milder deformities [56].

In patients with kyphotic deformities from ankylosing spondylitis where the cervical spine is rigidly fused, a posterior cervical extension osteotomy is a powerful technique for focal kyphosis correction. While there are various methods described, the generally accepted technique includes a standard prone positioning setup, followed by a posterior laminectomy, and resection of the C7-T1 facet joints. An opening wedge osteotomy preserves the pedicles and lengthens the anterior disc space while a closing wedge osteotomy generally requires some resection of the C7 pedicles in order to shorten the posterior column and not compress the exiting nerve roots. Upon completion of the osteotomy, the correction is obtained by head extension under close electrophysiological monitoring, with post-operative maintenance of correction by posterior instrumentation [57, 58].

A combination of both anterior and posterior approaches may be required in fixed deformities involving fusion of both the anterior and posterior spinal elements, when the required magnitude of correction cannot be achieved from a single approach alone, or for supplementing a long anterior fusion. There are a number of possible sequences of approaches, which can be undertaken. However, deciding the optimal approach depends on multiple factors, such as concurrent spinal cord compression, the presence and sites of bony fusion or instrumentation, and the magnitude of the kyphotic deformity [46].

Like any sequence starting anteriorly, an anterior-posterior-anterior approach can only be utilized if the deformity is not too severe (eg chin-on-chest-deformity) so as to allow for adequate visualization to permit access anteriorly without mobilizing the posteriorly fused segments. Although there are several variations, generally the first stage will comprise of an anterior corpectomy and uncinectomy, followed by a posterior instrumentation and appropriate (usually circumferential) osteotomies to permit for deformity correction, which is facilitated by applying a compressive force across the posterior instrumentation anchor sites. The patient is placed back into the supine position for the third stage, in which the interbody grafts are placed. By performing the anterior grafting as the final stage of the sequence, any potential graft loosening that may theoretically be displaced during the posterior osteotomy and corrective maneuvers can be visualized and addressed [9, 55].

However, approaching the anterior cervical spine a second time is usually associated with increased burden of post-operative challenges, such as significant edema of the soft tissue in the neck, which may compromise the patient's airway. In O'Shaughnessy's case series, the only patient who underwent the anterior-posterior-anterior sequence required both a gastrostomy and tracheostomy post-operatively, the authors partly attributed these complications to the extensive anterior dissection, which caused significant stretch on the esophagus and other surrounding neck structures [46]. Choosing this particular order of surgical approaches over the less morbid anterior-posterior sequence solely for the purpose of addressing a theoretical risk of anterior graft migration may not justify incurring the documented airway complications.

The posterior-anterior approach is appropriate when ankylosis is present in the posterior spinal column only and is not recommended if there remains any significant presence of anterior fusion. The first stage involves dorsal instrumentation and osteotomies for correction of the deformity, which is subsequently followed by a placement of an anterior interbody graft to allow for load sharing across the anterior column, thereby re-establishing the load-bearing abilities of the spine. There may be small osseous connections anteriorly, which can be indirectly released with corrective maneuvers following dorsal osteotomies [9, 46].

The posterior-anterior-posterior sequence can be utilized in the presence of posterior ankylosis and when a single approach is unable to provide adequate magnitude of correction. An initial stage of posterior releases, including laminectomies, facet osteotomies, Smith-Petersen osteotomies, as well as placement of posterior instrumentation (without rods) is accomplished to provide some initial deformity correction. The second procedure is comprised of multilevel anterior discectomies or disc osteotomies, interbody graft placement, and anterior plate fixation, either rigidly plated or simply to prevent anterior graft migration. Finally, the patient is turned back prone for the third stage, in which the posterior rods are placed to maintain the reduced position, in addition to performing fusions [9, 46]. Figure 6 demonstrates an illustrative depiction of the three stages and their respective components. The circumferential osteotomies and subsequent reconstructions permitted by the multi-sequence approach have yielded higher fusion rates. Therefore, patients with extensive spinal ankylosis or those at risk for pseudoarthrosis or structural compromise, may best be managed by a circumferential approach for optimal results [46].

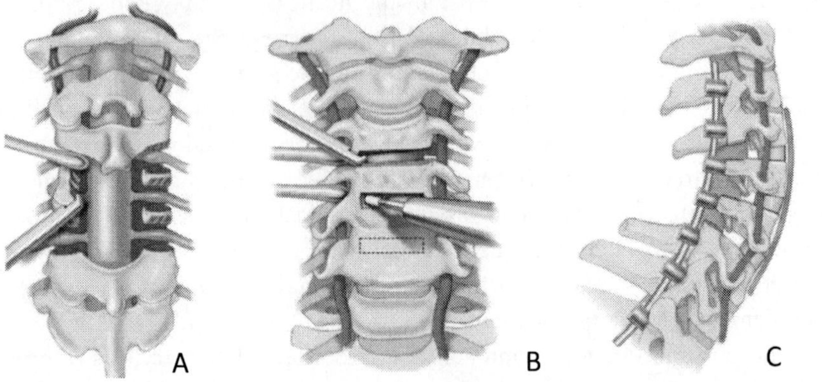

Figure 6. A 3-stage (posterior-anterior-posterior) approach with initial posterior decompression, corrective osteotomies, and screw insertion (A), followed by a 2nd stage through an anterior approach with multi-level osteotomies and discectomies (B). The final stage re-visits the spine posteriorly and places the rods through the prior instrumentations (C). (From Scheer JK, et al. Assessment and Treatment of Cervical Deformity. Neurosurg Clin N Am 2013, 24, 249-274., with permission).

Generally, the surgical correction is centered over the apex of the deformity and is expanded to a minimum of two levels in both the cephalad and caudal direction. For severe deformities requiring staged surgical approaches involving the upper subaxial cervical spine, we typically span the instrumentation levels from C2 down distally to the upper thoracic spine. We preferentially try to include C2 in our fixation as deemed appropriate, as the placement of pars or pedicle screws provides a significant biomechanical advantage for a rigid cephalad fixation point for our construct. For similar reasons, we also prefer spanning the cervicothoracic junction for lower subaxial deformities in favor of obtaining a more rigid construct with thoracic pedicle screws [9].

Fixed deformities, which are defined as the presence of ankylosis of one or more aspects of the spine leading to a postural rigidity, necessitate osteotomies to free up the fused regions. In releasing the anklyosed elements, a fixed deformity is effectively converted into a flexible deformity. The choice and type of osteotomy depends on the location and extent of the kyphosis. Sites of anterior ankylosis are generally treated with a combined anterior-posterior approach with anterior disc space osteotomies and posterior fusion, whereas in the presence of posterior ankylosis, a posterior-anterior-posterior approach comprised of posterior facet osteotomies, instrumentation and decompression, followed by anterior interbody graft placement, and final posterior instrumented fusion is pursued. Deformities centered at the cervicothoracic junction, especially those with circumferential ankylosis, usually require a posterior approach with posterior element or three-column (pedicle subtraction) osteotomy at C7 or in the upper thoracic spine [59].

The Smith Peterson osteotomy (SPO) was initially described in 1945 for addressing kyphotic deformities in patients with ankylosing spondylitis or rheumatoid arthritis [60-62]. However, its use has been expanded to include correction of Scheuermann's kyphosis, post-surgical iatrogenic sagittal imbalance, especially in the presence of fusion/malunion, and for any semirigid/rigid deformities of the cervical spine in the absence of anterior ankylosis [12, 63].

The SPO is essentially a posterior closing wedge osteotomy, in which the facets are removed posteriorly so as to allow the posterior elements of the cephalad spine to shorten the posterior column by closing down over a mobile disc space. As long as the disc space is mobile anteriorly or has the ability to open, the SPO is an effective corrective osteotomy. Specifically in patients with ankylosing spondylitis, the ankylosed disc space can open with posterior closure by rupture and osteoclasis of the ossified annulus. In comparison to a pedicle subtraction osteotomy, the SPO will confer relatively less correction (10.7 degrees per segment for SPO compared to 31.7 degrees for a single level pedicle subtraction osteotomy) and thus, additional successive SPOs at adjacent levels may be needed for correction of larger magnitude deformities [50, 63].

The pedicle subtraction osteotomy (PSO) was described for use in fixed sagittal deformities for both patients with ankylosing spondylitis and for rigid iatrogenic deformities [64-67]. In addressing cervical deformity, a PSO at the cervicothoracic junction (C7 or T1) typically minimizes injury to the vertebral arteries [57, 58, 68-71]. Other advantages of a cervicothoracic PSO includes the wider dimensions of the spinal canal at this level and the ability to preserve function of the upper extremity in the case of an iatrogenic injury to the spinal cord [25].

Pre-operative CT angiography is recommended to rule out aberrant anatomic variations of the vertebral artery at the C7 level. However, should a focal apex of extreme flexion deformity be present cephalad to the C7 level, the PSO can still be applied for attaining deformity correction. As the vertebral artery enters through the transverse foramen starting from the C6 level, a more extensive dissection will be necessary to expose both vertebral arteries from their respective foramen to ensure there is no vascular injury or kinking after the corrective maneuver [25, 26, 72].

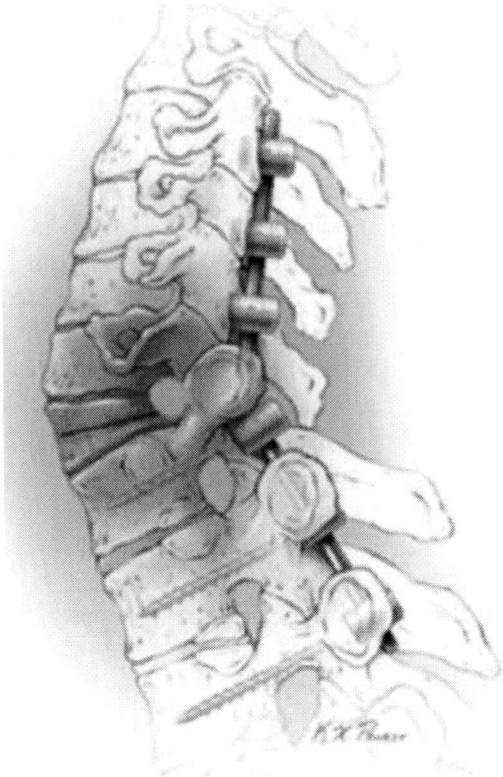

Figure 7. Pedicle subtraction osteotomy for correction of kyphotic deformities. (From Scheer JK, Tang JA, et al. Biomechanical analysis of osteotomy type and rod diameter for treatment of cervicothoracic kyphosis. Spine (Phila Pa 1976) 2011,36:E519-213, with permission.)

The PSO osteotomy is performed by a complete removal of the facets from C6-T1. The C7 and C8 nerve roots are then identified and protected and the C7 pedicle is isolated, skeletonized, and subsequently removed. Then, the C7 vertebral body is decancellated with spinal taps through the pedicle remnant site, as described by Deviren et al., after which angled currettes are utilized on both sides to further decancellate the vertebral body toward the midline to join the tapped holes. The lateral wall of the C7 vertebral body is dissected out and controlled removal with a needle-nose rongeur in piece-meal fashion with removal of the posterior body wall follows for completion of the osteotomy. The head holder is then loosened while the surgeon holds the head and carefully extends the neck for closure and subsequent correction. The head holder is tightened and rods are used to maintain the correction. The use of cobalt-chrome rods is preferred due to concerns of subsequent hardware failure, especially for significant deformity cases requiring larger constructs [27, 40].

In comparing the PSO with the SPO, several inherent properties of the PSO confer it significant biomechanical advantages in relation to the SPO. The SPO commonly involves either a disruption of the disc or osteoclasis through an anklyosed disc space during correction, which comprises the structural integrity of the anterior column. This results in gapping anteriorly due to tearing of the anterior longitudinal ligament, which is otherwise preserved in PSO. Furthermore, once the correction is obtained after a PSO, the significantly greater osseous contact affords stability across a wide load-sharing platform spanning all three spinal columns, which is depicted in Figure 7 [40, 73, 74].

The overall post-operative complication rate after cervical kyphosis correction varies significantly, ranging from 3.1% to as high as 34% [75, 76]. The incidence and type of complications will depend on the surgical approach, patient profile, and the surgical technique involved. The list of potential complications listed in the literature is lengthy, but fortunately permanently disabling complications, such as spinal cord injury, and mortalities are relatively low. Acute complications arising from intra-operative causes include displacement of the implant or graft, dysphagia, infection, dural tears, neurologic deficits, vertebral artery injury, hoarseness of voice, and dyspnea. Subsequent complications can include pseudoarthrosis, hardware failure with resultant progression of the deformity, pulmonary embolism, deep venous thrombosis, pneumonia, and post-operative hematoma [9, 46, 75-77] [27, 55].

Grosso et al. followed 19 patients who underwent various surgical approaches (anterior, posterior, and combined) for correction of cervical kyphosis, in which 26 complications were reported [76]. The most common complications, in order of decreasing incidence, were deep vein thrombosis, deep wound infection, pneumonia, pulmonary embolism, hematoma, followed by prolonged dysphagia requiring placement of a feeding tube [76]. Patients who had a combined anterior and posterior approach demonstrated a higher incidence of complications than either of the single approaches (40% for combined, 30% for anterior, 27% for posterior), although the amount of surgical correction was similar across the various approaches [76]. Mortality was a relatively uncommon complication (4%), with the causes of death comprised of sepsis, epidural hematoma, and as a late sequela from a perforated megacolon [76]. Although the anterior only approach showed similar correction but a lower rate of complication than the combined approach, the utility of the combined approach should still not be underestimated, as it has shown higher fusion rates for patients at higher risk of non-union [76]. For example, neurofibromatosis patients undergoing correction by either a single posterior approach versus a combined approach were assessed in multiple studies, all of which showed significantly higher failure rate in the posterior approach alone (53% failure in posterior versus 23% in the combined for a series of 56 patients) [68, 78-81].

Post-operative neurologic deficits, while relatively common, are usually transient and will resolve spontaneously with time. In O'Shaughnessy's series of 16 patients treated for post-laminectomy kyphosis with circumferential osteotomy and instrumented fusion, three patients (19%) demonstrated a C5 palsy [46]. A meta-analysis on 183 patients with ankylosing spondylitis who underwent surgical correction of cervical kyphosis demonstrated a 19% incidence of C8 palsy [25]. Permanent neurologic deficits, while rare, were still reported however. O'Shaughnessy reported one patient with quadriplegia from failure of the head-holder, while the meta-analysis on ankylosing spondylitis cervical kyphosis patients showed 5 of 183 patients (3%) with permanent spinal cord injury [9, 46, 57, 68, 71].

Respiratory and swallowing difficulty post-operatively were more common after anterior approaches, especially in the multi-stage sequences requiring revisiting the anterior spine and those associated with larger surgical exposures and lengthier operative durations. Conversely, placing surgical drains, paying attention to hemostasis intra-operatively, and keeping patients intubated if there is concern for significant anterior cervical edema can reduce the incidence of such complications. Postoperative dysphagia usually resolved within weeks [9, 57, 58, 77].

Postoperative Care

Especially for patients with significant corrective surgery or with multiple approaches necessitating a staged approach, a post-operative admission to the intensive care unit is commonplace. For multi-stage procedures spanning over several days, keeping the patient intubated in between stages should be considered, as it addresses the potential complication of a difficult airway due to significant facial and anterior cervical edema. In posterior-anterior-posterior approaches spanning several days, we recommend obtaining a CT scans prior to the final stage to confirm appropriate screw placement and allow for screw redirection if necessary. Some authors have recommend insertion of a temporary nasoduodenal feeding tube postoperatively or between stages [46].

Upon completion of the procedures and post-extubation, patients should undergo swallow evaluation to rule out swallowing disorders before advancing the diet. Enteral nutrition is initiated through a nasoduodenal tube for patients who have impaired swallowing. If swallowing dysfunction persists beyond 7-10 days, a percutaneous gastrostomy tube can be considered. Patients with persistent post-operative dyspnea or excessive secretions may require a tracheostomy [9, 46].

All patients will initially be immobilized in a rigid cervical collar for 6-12 weeks. For more unstable or extensive corrections requiring further support, a temporary halo-vest orthosis can also be considered.

Summary

Patients with cervical kyphosis can present with loss of horizontal gaze, neck pain, postural instability and possibly neurologic deficits. An important debilitating aspect of its natural history is its propensity to worsen over time as kyphotic collapse results in an anterior shift of the weight-bearing axis. The etiologies of cervical kyphosis are diverse, however, a similar approach to evaluation and management can be undertaken.

Patients with cervical kyphosis should undergo a thorough physical examination that includes assessment of the severity of the deformity, relative flexibility as well as any associated neurologic deficits. The severity of the deformity can be further quantified using radiographic parameters estimated using plain radiography. CT imaging or MRI remains useful adjuncts for preoperative surgical planning.

Although mild cervical kyphosis can be managed with non-operative treatment, symptomatically severe deformity requires surgical intervention. The principles of surgical management include correction of alignment, possible decompression of neural elements, and restoration of sagittal balance. Generally, surgical decision-making includes selection of approach (anterior, posterior or both) and method of deformity correction, which may involve shortening of the posterior column, lengthening of the anterior column or a combination of both methods. Careful attention to complication avoidance, such as dysphagia, airway compromise, is critical.

Cervical kyphosis remains a challenging and complex pathology that requires a comprehensive understanding of its pathoanatomy as well as appreciation of the diverse set of etiologies that can contribute to this deformity. Appropriate evaluation, imaging, selection of surgical treatment strategies and postoperative care are the critical elements of optimal management.

Illustrative Clinical Cases

Case 1

71 year-old female with progressive kyphotic deformity of the cervical spine with dropped head syndrome who failed extensive physical therapy and bracing and found to have flexible focal cervical kyphosis (Figure 8 and Figure 9). She underwent a single stage anterior approach for a 2-level fusion with cage prosthesis. Correction of the deformity was obtained with placement of interbody structural allografts and anterior plating without necessitating corrective osteotomies (Figure 10).

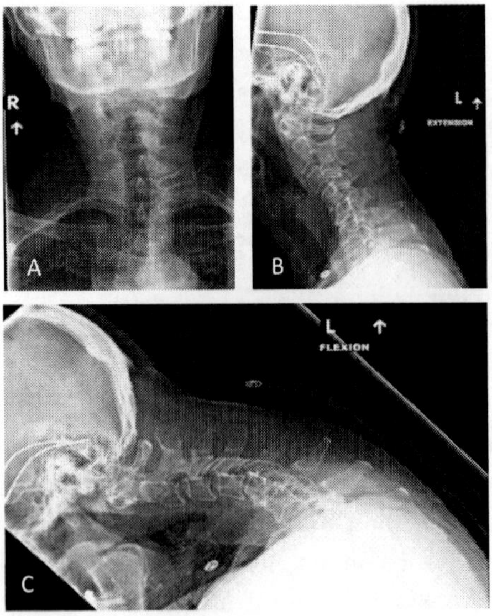

Figure 8. Case 1. Pre-operative cervical spine plain radiographs AP (A), Lateral Extension (B) Lateral Flexion (C) demonstrating flexible kyphotic apex at C4-C5 which did not fully reduce with extension.

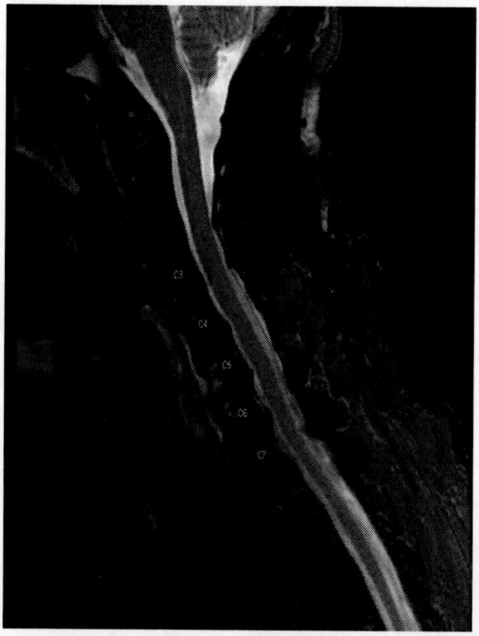

Figure 9. Case 1. MRI T2 imaging of cervical spine.

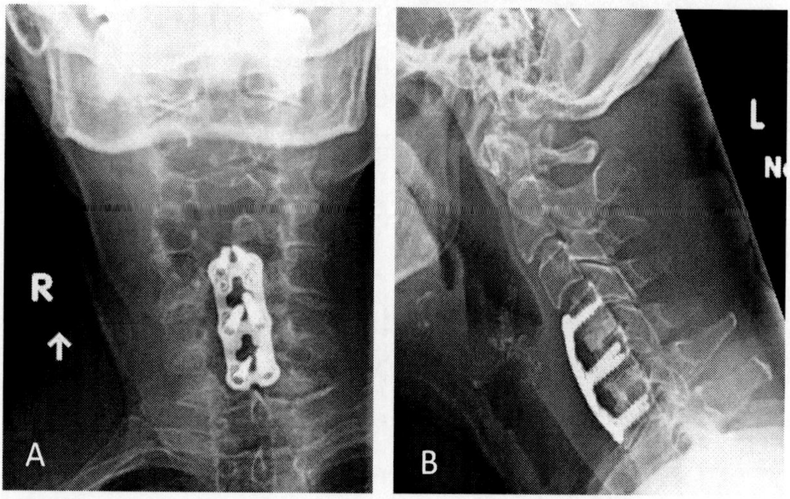

Figure 10. Case 1. Post-operative radiographs AP (A) and Lateral (B) with C4-C6 anterior cervical fusion, interbody structural allograft insertion, and anterior plate instrumentation with lordotic restoration.

Case 2

51 year-old female with history of multiple prior failed cervical and lumbar surgeries, including an unsuccessful prior anterior fusion at C4-C6 and instrumentation failure at C4-C5, who presented with cervical myelopathy, progressive paresthesia, weakness, and gait abnormalities in association with a fixed lumbar kyphosis. Pre-operative radiographs demonstrated C3-C4 spondylolisthesis with severe stenosis, in addition to cervical kyphosis (Figure 11 and Figure 12). She underwent a C4 corpectomy, interbody fusions of C6-7 and C7-T1 and anterior plating from C4-T1 followed by a posterior C2-T3 instrumented fusion. Postoperative images and clinical picture demonstrated improvement in sagittal balance and horizontal gaze (Figure 13).

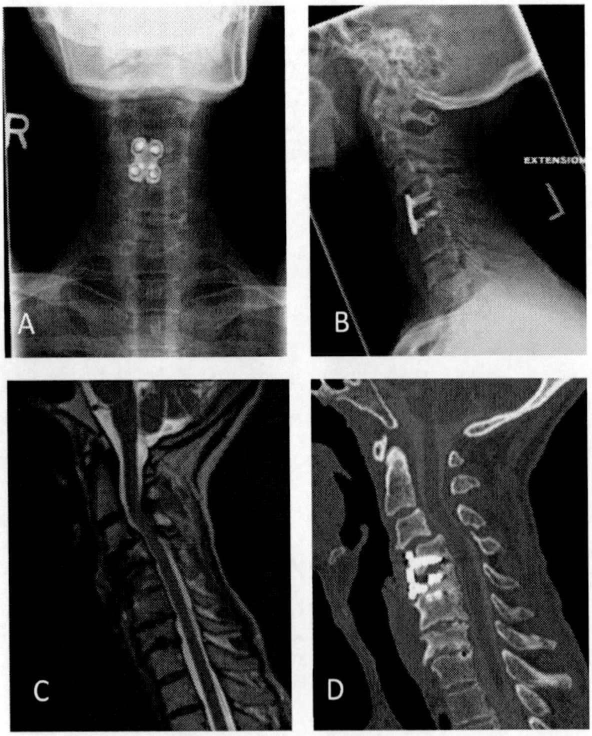

Figure 11. Case 2. Pre-operative radiographs AP (A) and Lateral (B) and MRI T2 imaging (C) and CT imaging (D) demonstrating multi-level stenosis, pseudoarthrosis, and broken instrumentation.

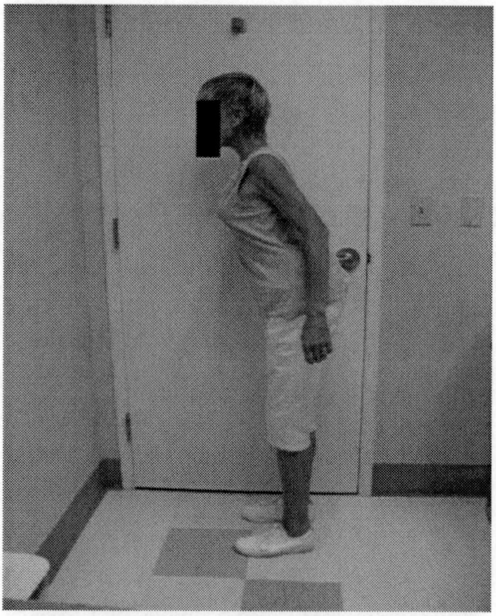

Figure 12. Case 2. Preoperative clinical picture demonstrating loss of sagittal balance.

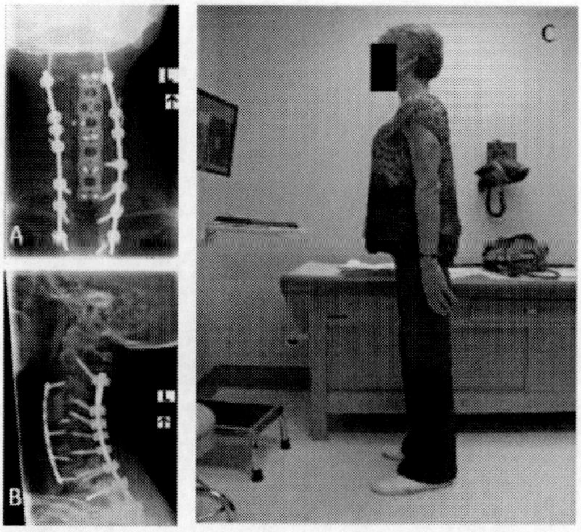

Figure 13. Case 2. Patient underwent a C4 corpectomy, interbody grafts at C6-7 and C7-T1 with anterior plating from C3-T1 followed by posterior instrumented fusion from C2 to T3. Postoperative radiographs AP (A) and Lateral (B). Post-operative clinical photograph demonstrate improvement of sagittal balance (C).

Case 3

80 year-old male with a fixed post-laminectomy kyphotic deformity with resultant chin-on-chest deformity as shown on plain radiography and CT imaging (Figure 14 and Figure 15) with progressive cervical myelopathy with pre-operative MRI showing signal cord changes and the spinal cord draped over the vertebral bodies (Figure 16).

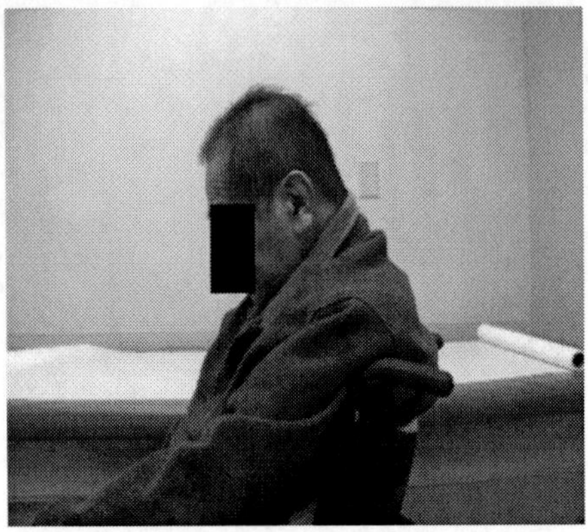

Figure 14. Case 3. Clinical photograph demonstrated kyphosis with chin-on-chest deformity.

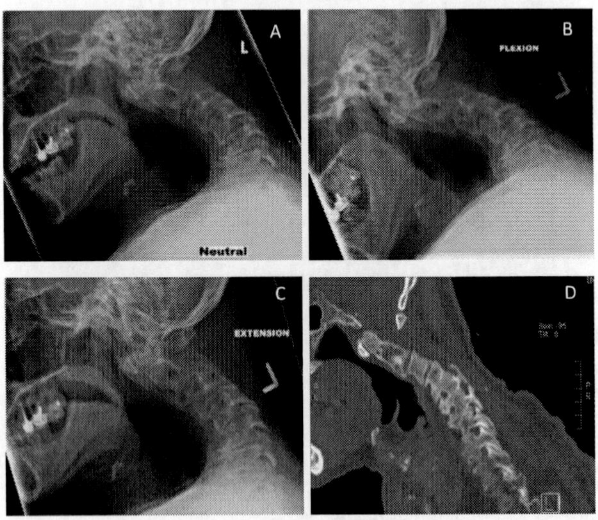

Figure 15. Case 3. Pre-operative radiographs Lateral Neutral (A), Lateral Flexion (B), Lateral Extension (C), and CT imaging (D) demonstrating rigid cervical kyphosis.

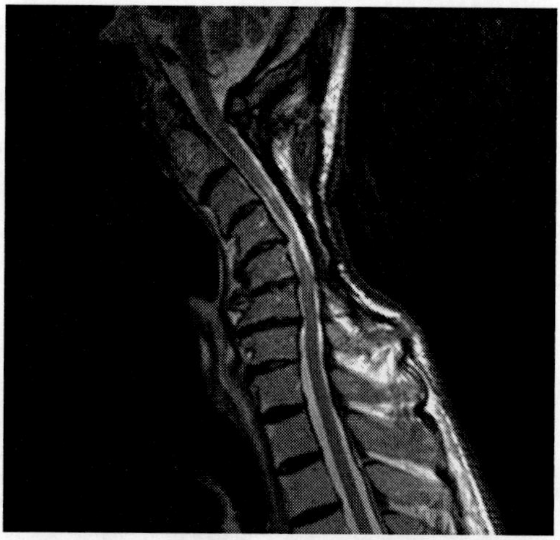

Figure 16. Case 3. Pre-operative MRI T2 imaging of cervical spine.

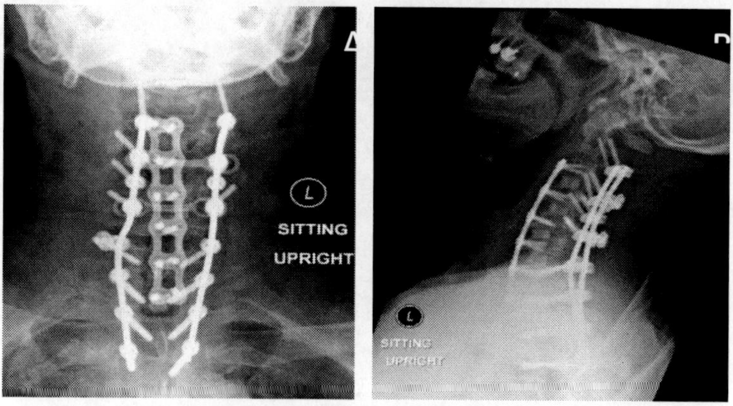

Figure 17. Case 3. *First stage* instrumentation included C2-T3 instrumentation with facet osteotomies, after which C3-CT1 anterior diskectomies and partial corpectomies of C6 and C7 were done during the *2nd stage*, an anterior plate was also placed during this time after interbody graft placement and fusion from C3 to T1.After the majority of the correction was achieved during the 2nd stage, the *final stage* involved rod insertion from C2-T3 posteriorly and fusion to secure the lordotic alignment. Final radiographs AP (A) and Lateral (B).

A three-stage posterior-anterior-posterior approach, with an initial posterior instrumentation and decompression, corrective osteotomy and instrumentation was then followed by a 2nd stage anterior multi-level cervical discectomy with interbody restoration for lordotic correction, followed by a final posterior rod insertion and fusion (Figure 17). Post-operatively, the patient's horizontal gaze was restored and myelopathy improved.

Case 4

19 year-old male with Scheuermann's kyphosis with extensive prior surgical corrective history, including Smith-Peterson osteotomies at T1 and T2, posterior thoracic instrumented fusion, presents with worsening proximal junctional kyphosis with chin-on-chest deformity centered over the cervicothoracic junction with difficulty obtaining horizontal gaze (Figure 18 and Figure 19).

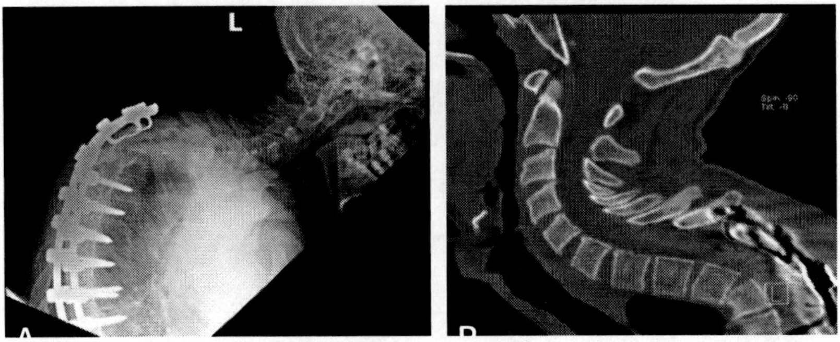

Figure 18. Case 4. Pre-operative radiographs Lateral (A) and CT imaging (B) demonstrating proximal junctional kyphosis centered over the cervicothoracic junction.

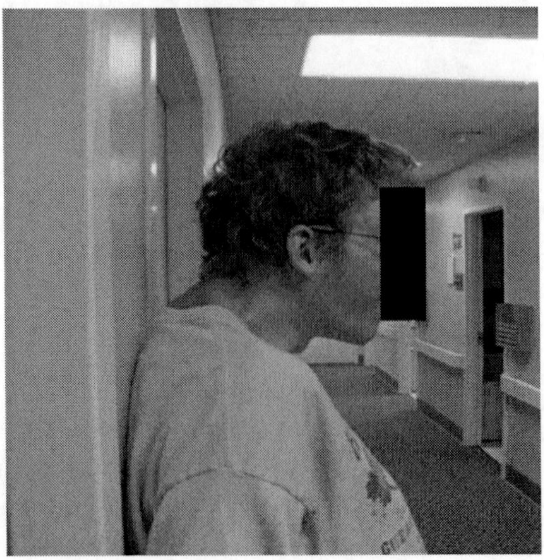

Figure 19. Case 4. Pre-operative clinic photograph demonstrating cervical kyphosis.

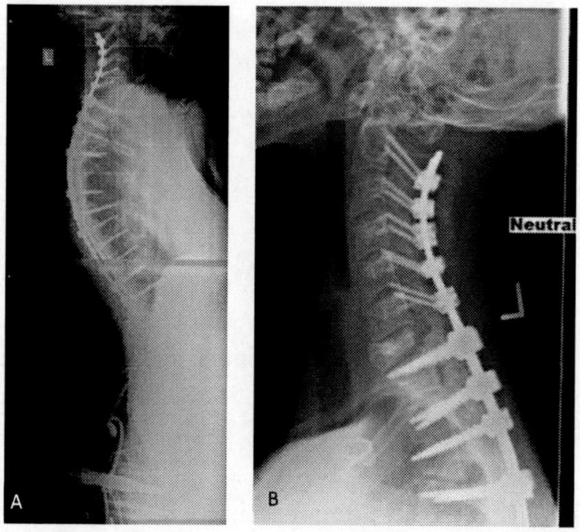

Figure 20. Case 4. After undergoing a C7 pedicle subtraction osteotomy and C2-T12 posterior instrumented fusion, patient had full correction in the sagittal plane with restoration of horizontal gaze, as depicted on postoperative radiographs Full-length Lateral (A) and lateral cervical spine (B).

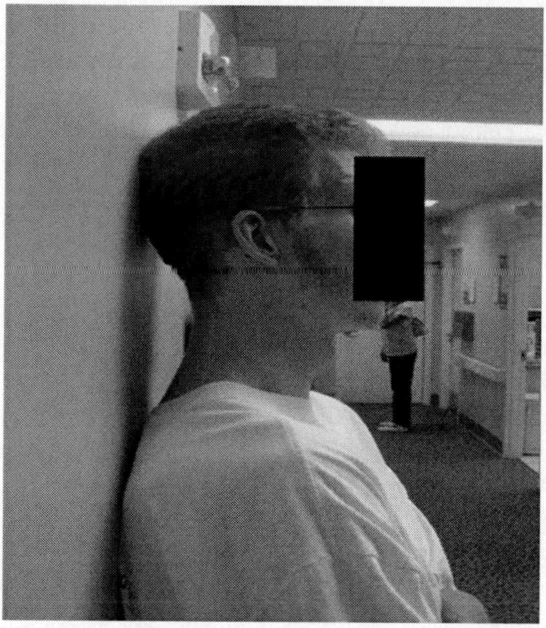

Figure 21. Case 4. Postoperative clinical picture demonstrating restoration of cervical sagittal alignment.

Patient underwent hardware removal, pedicle subtraction osteotomy at C7, with C2-T12 instrumentation (Figure 20). Postoperative clinical picture demonstrated the improvement in kyphosis attributed to the single level (Figure 21).

References

[1] Hoy, DG, Protani, M, De, R, Buchbinder, R. The epidemiology of neck pain. *Best Pract Res Clin Rheumatol*, 2010, 24, 783-92.

[2] Cohen, SP. Epidemiology, diagnosis, and treatment of neck pain. *Mayo Clin Proc*, 2015, 90, 284-99.

[3] Salemi, G, Savettieri, G, Meneghini, F, et al. Prevalence of cervical spondylotic radiculopathy: a door-to-door survey in a Sicilian municipality. *Acta Neurol Scand*, 1996, 93, 184-8.

[4] Radhakrishnan, K, Litchy, WJ, O'Fallon, WM, Kurland, LT. Epidemiology of cervical radiculopathy. A population-based study from Rochester, Minnesota, 1976 through 1990. *Brain*, 1994, 117 (Pt 2), 325-35.

[5] Le, Huec, JC, Demezon, H, Aunoble, S. Sagittal parameters of global cervical balance using EOS imaging: normative values from a prospective cohort of asymptomatic volunteers. *Eur Spine J*, 2015, 24, 63-71.

[6] Glassman, SD, Berven, S, Bridwell, K, Horton, W, Dimar, JR. Correlation of radiographic parameters and clinical symptoms in adult scoliosis. *Spine* (Phila Pa 1976), 2005, 30, 682-8.

[7] Glassman, SD, Bridwell, K, Dimar, JR, Horton, W, Berven, S, Schwab, F. The impact of positive sagittal balance in adult spinal deformity. *Spine* (Phila Pa 1976), 2005, 30, 2024-9.

[8] Tang, JA, Scheer, JK, Smith, JS, et al. The impact of standing regional cervical sagittal alignment on outcomes in posterior cervical fusion surgery. *Neurosurgery*, 2012, 71, 662-9, discussion 9.

[9] Han, K, Lu, C, Li, J, et al. Surgical treatment of cervical kyphosis. *Eur Spine J*, 2011, 20, 523-36.

[10] Iwasaki, M, Yamamoto, T, Miyauchi, A, Amano, K, Yonenobu, K. Cervical kyphosis: predictive factors for progression of kyphosis and myelopathy. *Spine* (Phila Pa 1976), 2002, 27, 1419-25.

[11] Winestone, JS, Farley, CW, Curt, BA, et al. Laminectomy, durotomy, and piotomy effects on spinal cord intramedullary pressure in severe cervical and thoracic kyphotic deformity: a cadaveric study. *J Neurosurg Spine*, 2012, 16, 195-200.

[12] Scheer, JK, Tang, JA, Smith JS, et al. Cervical spine alignment, sagittal deformity, and clinical implications: a review. *J Neurosurg Spine*, 2013, 19, 141-59.

[13] Albert, TJ, Vacarro, A. Postlaminectomy kyphosis. *Spine* (Phila Pa 1976), 1998, 23, 2738-45.

[14] Kaptain, GJ, Simmons, NE, Replogle, RE, Pobereskin, L. Incidence and outcome of kyphotic deformity following laminectomy for cervical spondylotic myelopathy. *J Neurosurg*, 2000, 93, 199-204.

[15] Guigui, P, Benoist, M, Deburge A. Spinal deformity and instability after multilevel cervical laminectomy for spondylotic myelopathy. *Spine* (Phila Pa 1976), 1998, 23, 440-7.

[16] Suk, KS, Kim, KT, Lee, JH, Lee, SH, Lim, YJ, Kim, JS. Sagittal alignment of the cervical spine after the laminoplasty. *Spine* (Phila Pa 1976), 2007, 32, E656-60.

[17] Bell, DF, Walker, JL, O'Connor, G, Tibshirani, R. Spinal deformity after multiple-level cervical laminectomy in children. *Spine* (Phila Pa 1976), 1994, 19, 406-11.

[18] Yasuoka, S, Peterson, HA, MacCarty, CS. Incidence of spinal column deformity after multilevel laminectomy in children and adults. *J Neurosurg*, 1982, 57, 441-5.

[19] Tsirikos, AI, Saifuddin, A, Noordeen, MH. Spinal deformity in neurofibromatosis type-1: diagnosis and treatment. *Eur Spine J*, 2005, 14, 427-39.

[20] Kokubun, S, Ozawa, H, Sakurai, M, Ishii, Y. One-stage anterior and posterior correction of severe kyphosis of the cervical spine in neurofibromatosis. A case report. *Spine* (Phila Pa 1976), 1993, 18, 2332-5.

[21] Nijland, EA, van den Berg, MP, Wuisman, PI, van Royen, BJ, Winters, HA, van Ouwerkerk, WJ. Correction of a dystrophic cervicothoracic spine deformity in Recklinghausen's disease. *Clin Orthop Relat Res*, 1998, 149-55.

[22] Yong-Hing, K, Kalamchi, A, MacEwen, GD. Cervical spine abnormalities in neurofibromatosis. *J Bone Joint Surg Am*, 1979, 61, 695-9.

[23] Kawabata, S, Watanabe, K, Hosogane, N, et al. Surgical correction of severe cervical kyphosis in patients with neurofibromatosis Type 1. *J Neurosurg Spine*, 2013, 18, 274-9.

[24] Ma, J, Wu, Z, Yang, X, Xiao, J. Surgical treatment of severe cervical dystrophic kyphosis due to neurofibromatosis Type 1: a review of 8 cases. *J Neurosurg Spine*, 2011, 14, 93-8.

[25] Hoh, DJ, Khoueir, P, Wang, MY. Management of cervical deformity in ankylosing spondylitis. *Neurosurg Focus*, 2008, 24, E9.

[26] Mummaneni, PV, Mummaneni, VP, Haid, RW. Jr, Rodts, GE, Jr, Sasso, RC. Cervical osteotomy for the correction of chin-on-chest deformity in ankylosing spondylitis. Technical note. Neurosurg Focus 2003, 14:e9.

[27] Deviren, V, Scheer, JK, Ames, CP. Technique of cervicothoracic junction pedicle subtraction osteotomy for cervical sagittal imbalance: report of 11 cases. *J Neurosurg Spine*, 2011, 15, 174-81.

[28] Kim, KT, Lee, SH, Son, ES, Kwack, YH, Chun, YS, Lee, JH. Surgical treatment of "chin-on-pubis" deformity in a patient with ankylosing spondylitis: a case report of consecutive cervical, thoracic, and lumbar corrective osteotomies. *Spine* (Phila Pa 1976), 2012, 37, E1017-21.

[29] Kim, KT, Suk, KS, Cho, YJ, Hong, GP, Park, BJ. Clinical outcome results of pedicle subtraction osteotomy in ankylosing spondylitis with kyphotic deformity. *Spine* (Phila Pa 1976), 2002, 27, 612-8.

[30] Wang, Y, Zhang, Y, Mao, K, et al. Transpedicular bivertebrae wedge osteotomy and discectomy in lumbar spine for severe ankylosing spondylitis. *J Spinal Disord Tech*, 2010, 23, 186-91.

[31] Rajasekaran, S. Kyphotic deformity in spinal tuberculosis and its management. *Int Orthop*, 2012, 36, 359-65.

[32] Yusof, MI, Hassan, E, Rahmat, N, Yunus, R. Spinal tuberculosis: the association between pedicle involvement and anterior column damage and kyphotic deformity. *Spine* (Phila Pa 1976), 2009, 34, 713-7.

[33] Takahashi, H, Yokoyama, Y, Terajima, F, et al. Isolated neck extensor myopathy causing a dropped head: a case report. *J Orthop Surg (Hong Kong)*, 2011, 19, 104-7.

[34] Kashihara, K, Ohno, M, Tomita, S. Dropped head syndrome in Parkinson's disease. *Mov Disord*, 2006, 21, 1213-6.

[35] Katz, JS, Wolfe, GI, Burns, DK, Bryan, WW, Fleckenstein, JL, Barohn, RJ. Isolated neck extensor myopathy: a common cause of dropped head syndrome. *Neurology*, 1996, 46, 917-21.

[36] Chi, JH, Tay, B, Stahl, D, Lee, R. Complex deformities of the cervical spine. *Neurosurg Clin N Am*, 2007, 18, 295-304.

[37] Mummaneni, PV, Deutsch, H, Mummaneni, VP. Cervicothoracic kyphosis. *Neurosurg Clin N Am*, 2006, 17, 277-87, vi.

[38] Pigge, RR, Scheerder, FJ, Smit, TH, Mullender, MG, van Royen, BJ. Effectiveness of preoperative planning in the restoration of balance and view in ankylosing spondylitis. *Neurosurg Focus*, 2008, 24, E7.

[39] Suk, KS, Kim, KT, Lee, SH, Kim, JM. Significance of chin-brow vertical angle in correction of kyphotic deformity of ankylosing spondylitis patients. *Spine* (Phila Pa 1976), 2003, 28, 2001-5.

[40] Scheer, JK, Ames, CP, Deviren, V. Assessment and treatment of cervical deformity. *Neurosurg Clin N Am*, 2013, 24, 249-74.

[41] Harrison, DE, Harrison, DD, Cailliet, R, Troyanovich, SJ, Janik, TJ, Holland, B. Cobb method or Harrison posterior tangent method: which to choose for lateral cervical radiographic analysis. *Spine* (Phila Pa 1976), 2000, 25, 2072-8.

[42] Polly, DW, Jr, Kilkelly, FX, McHale, KA, Asplund, LM, Mulligan, M, Chang, AS. Measurement of lumbar lordosis. Evaluation of intraobserver, interobserver, and technique variability. *Spine* (Phila Pa 1976), 1996, 21, 1530-5, discussion 5-6.

[43] Singer, KP, Jones, TJ, Breidahl, PD. A comparison of radiographic and computer-assisted measurements of thoracic and thoracolumbar sagittal curvature. *Skeletal Radiol*, 1990, 19, 21-6.

[44] Lee, SH, Kim, KT, Seo, EM, Suk, KS, Kwack, YH, Son ES. The influence of thoracic inlet al.ignment on the craniocervical sagittal balance in asymptomatic adults. *J Spinal Disord Tech*, 2012, 25, E41-7.

[45] Steinmetz, MP, Stewart, TJ, Kager, CD, Benzel, EC, Vaccaro, AR. Cervical deformity correction. *Neurosurgery*, 2007, 60, S90-7.

[46] O'Shaughnessy, BA, Liu, JC, Hsieh, PC, Koski, TR, Ganju, A, Ondra, SL. Surgical treatment of fixed cervical kyphosis with myelopathy. *Spine* (Phila Pa 1976), 2008, 33, 771-8.

[47] Ferch, RD, Shad, A, Cadoux-Hudson, TA, Teddy, PJ. Anterior correction of cervical kyphotic deformity: effects on myelopathy, neck pain, and sagittal alignment. *J Neurosurg*, 2004, 100, 13-9.

[48] Herman, JM, Sonntag, VK. Cervical corpectomy and plate fixation for postlaminectomy kyphosis. *J Neurosurg*, 1994, 80, 963-70.

[49] Steinmetz, MP, Kager, CD, Benzel, EC. Ventral correction of postsurgical cervical kyphosis. *J Neurosurg*, 2003, 98, 1-7.

[50] Cho, KJ, Bridwell, KH, Lenke, LG, Berra, A, Baldus, C. Comparison of Smith-Petersen versus pedicle subtraction osteotomy for the correction

of fixed sagittal imbalance. *Spine* (Phila Pa 1976), 2005, 30, 2030-7, discussion 8.

[51] Ames CP, Blondel B, Scheer JK, et al. Cervical radiographical alignment: comprehensive assessment techniques and potential importance in cervical myelopathy. Spine (Phila Pa 1976), 2013, 38, S149-60.

[52] Stewart, TJ, Steinmetz, MP, Benzel, EC. Techniques for the ventral correction of postsurgical cervical kyphotic deformity. *Neurosurgery*, 2005, 56, 191-5, discussion -5.

[53] Liu, Y, Chen, Y, Yang, L, et al. The surgical treatment and related management for post-tubercular kyphotic deformity of the cervical spine or the cervico-thoracic spine. *Int Orthop*, 2012, 36, 367-72.

[54] Park, Y, Riew, KD, Cho, W. The long-term results of anterior surgical reconstruction in patients with postlaminectomy cervical kyphosis. *Spine J*, 2010, 10, 380-7.

[55] Abumi, K, Shono, Y, Taneichi, H, Ito, M, Kaneda, K. Correction of cervical kyphosis using pedicle screw fixation systems. *Spine* (Phila Pa 1976), 1999, 24, 2389-96.

[56] Jones, EL, Heller, JG, Silcox, DH, Hutton, WC. Cervical pedicle screws versus lateral mass screws. Anatomic feasibility and biomechanical comparison. *Spine* (Phila Pa 1976), 1997, 22, 977-82.

[57] Belanger, TA, Milam, RAt, Roh, JS, Bohlman, HH. Cervicothoracic extension osteotomy for chin-on-chest deformity in ankylosing spondylitis. *J Bone Joint Surg Am*, 2005, 87, 1732-8.

[58] McMaster, MJ. Osteotomy of the cervical spine in ankylosing spondylitis. *J Bone Joint Surg Br*, 1997, 79, 197-203.

[59] Hann, S, Chalouhi, N, Madineni, R, et al. An algorithmic strategy for selecting a surgical approach in cervical deformity correction. *Neurosurg Focus*, 2014, 36, E5.

[60] Smith-Petersen, MN, Larson, CB, Aufranc, OE. Osteotomy of the spine for correction of flexion deformity in rheumatoid arthritis. *Clin Orthop Relat Res*, 1969, 66, 6-9.

[61] McMaster, MJ. A technique for lumbar spinal osteotomy in ankylosing spondylitis. *J Bone Joint Surg Br*, 1985, 67, 204-10.

[62] Kostuik, JP, Maurais, GR, Richardson, WJ, Okajima, Y. Combined single stage anterior and posterior osteotomy for correction of iatrogenic lumbar kyphosis. *Spine* (Phila Pa 1976), 1988, 13, 257-66.

[63] Bridwell, KH. Decision making regarding Smith-Petersen vs. pedicle subtraction osteotomy vs. vertebral column resection for spinal deformity. *Spine* (Phila Pa 1976), 2006, 31, S171-8.

[64] Thomasen, E. Vertebral osteotomy for correction of kyphosis in ankylosing spondylitis. *Clin Orthop Relat Res*, 1985, 142-52.

[65] Bridwell, KH, Lewis, SJ, Rinella, A, Lenke, LG, Baldus, C, Blanke, K. Pedicle subtraction osteotomy for the treatment of fixed sagittal imbalance. Surgical technique. *J Bone Joint Surg Am*, 2004, 86-A Suppl, 1, 44-50.

[66] Bridwell, KH, Lewis, SJ, Edwards, C, et al. Complications and outcomes of pedicle subtraction osteotomies for fixed sagittal imbalance. *Spine* (Phila Pa 1976) 2003, 28, 2093-101.

[67] Berven, SH, Deviren, V, Smith, JA, Emami, A, Hu, SS, Bradford, DS. Management of fixed sagittal plane deformity: results of the transpedicular wedge resection osteotomy. *Spine* (Phila Pa 1976), 2001, 26, 2036-43.

[68] Langeloo, DD, Journee, HL, Pavlov, PW, de Kleuver, M. Cervical osteotomy in ankylosing spondylitis: evaluation of new developments. *Eur Spine J*, 2006, 15, 493-500.

[69] Mehdian, SM, Freeman, BJ, Licina, P. Cervical osteotomy for ankylosing spondylitis: an innovative variation on an existing technique. *Eur Spine J*, 1999, 8, 505-9.

[70] Shimizu, K, Matsushita, M, Fujibayashi, S, Toguchida, J, Ido, K, Nakamura, T. Correction of kyphotic deformity of the cervical spine in ankylosing spondylitis using general anesthesia and internal fixation. *J Spinal Disord*, 1996, 9, 540-3.

[71] Simmons, ED, DiStefano, RJ, Zheng, Y, Simmons, EH. Thirty-six years experience of cervical extension osteotomy in ankylosing spondylitis: techniques and outcomes. *Spine* (Phila Pa 1976), 2006, 31, 3006-12.

[72] Duff, SE, Grundy, PL, Gill, SS. New approach to cervical flexion deformity in ankylosing spondylitis. Case report. *J Neurosurg*, 2000, 93, 283-6.

[73] Scheer, JK, Tang, JA, Buckley, JM, et al. Biomechanical analysis of osteotomy type and rod diameter for treatment of cervicothoracic kyphosis. *Spine* (Phila Pa 1976), 2011, 36, E519-23.

[74] Scheer, JK, Tang, JA, Deviren, V, et al. Biomechanical analysis of cervicothoracic junction osteotomy in cadaveric model of ankylosing spondylitis: effect of rod material and diameter. *J Neurosurg Spine*, 2011, 14, 330-5.

[75] Etame, AB, Wang, AC, Than, KD, La Marca, F, Park, P. Outcomes after surgery for cervical spine deformity: review of the literature. *Neurosurg Focus*, 2010, 28, E14.

[76] Grosso, MJ, Hwang, R, Krishnaney, AA, Mroz, TE, Benzel, EC, Steinmetz, MP. Complications and Outcomes for Surgical Approaches to Cervical Kyphosis. *J Spinal Disord Tech*, 2013.

[77] Sagi, HC, Beutler, W, Carroll, E, Connolly, PJ. Airway complications associated with surgery on the anterior cervical spine. *Spine*, (Phila Pa 1976) 2002, 27, 949-53.

[78] Parisini P, Di Silvestre M, Greggi T, Paderni S, Cervellati S, Savini R. Surgical correction of dystrophic spinal curves in neurofibromatosis. A review of 56 patients. *Spine* (Phila Pa 1976), 1999, 24, 2247-53.

[79] Sirois, JL, 3rd, Drennan, JC. Dystrophic spinal deformity in neurofibromatosis. *J Pediatr Orthop*, 1990, 10, 522-6.

[80] Winter, RB. Thoracic lordoscoliosis in neurofibromatosis: treatment by a Harrington rod with sublaminar wiring. Report of two cases. *J Bone Joint Surg Am*, 1984, 66, 1102-6.

[81] Winter, RB, Lonstein, JE, Anderson, M. Neurofibromatosis hyperkyphosis: a review of 33 patients with kyphosis of 80 degrees or greater. *J Spinal Disord*, 1988, 1, 39-49.

In: Kyphosis
Editor: Janice Newton

ISBN: 978-1-63483-224-3

Chapter IV

Scheuermann's Kyphosis

Marios G. Lykissas*[1,*]*, MD, PhD, Janina Kueper*[1]*, MD, Alexander Aichmair*[1]*, MD, and Ioannis Gkiatas*[2]*, MD

[1]Department of Orthopedic Surgery, Spine and Scoliosis Service, Hospital for Special Surgery, Weill Cornell Medical College, New York, NY, US

[2]Department of Orthopaedic Suegery, University Hospital of Ioannina, Ioannina, Greece

Abstract

Scheuermann's disease is a type of permanent structural kyphosis which develops in approximately 0.4 to 8.3% of the pre-adolescent population. The deformity is radiographically defined by the vertebral wedging of at least three adjacent vertebral bodies angled a minimum of 5°. The reported etiology and the incidence amongst sexes vary widely amongst studies. Scheuermann's kyphosis is histologically identified by the disorganized and defective endochondral ossification of vertebral end plates resulting in a disruption of growth. The biochemical dysbalance of the matrix components, collagen and mucopolysaccharide, render the vertebral end plate weak and vulnerable to mechanical strains, resulting in the pathognomonic vertebral wedging. Different hypotheses have been discussed as origins of the disorder. In fact, juvenile osteoporosis, the level of physical activity, weight and height, as well as sternum length and growth hormone levels have been discussed as potential contributing or causal factors of the disease. Great dissent in the scientific community exists to this day pertaining the degree of influence of genetics on the pathogenesis of the disease. Patients with Scheuermann's disease may present at a diverse range of age with complaints of pain, postural changes and rarely neurological or cardiopulmonary compromise. Upon clinical examination, patients will demonstrate excessive fixed kyphosis in the thoracic- or lumbar vertebrae with little or no correction on hyperextension. Non-structural compensatory features may also include pelvic anteversion, shoulder rounding and lumbar as well as cervical hyperlordosis. Radiographs of the spine demonstrate kyphotic deformity in the thoracic, thoracolumbar or lumbar vertebrae associated with vertebral wedging and disk space narrowing between the angulated vertebrae. Additional typical features which may be found are end plate irregularities and intraosseous disk herniations, also referred to as Schmorl nodes. The management of Scheuermann's disease has traditionally been focused on conservative measures such as observation, symptomatic pain relief, physical therapy and rehabilitation as well as bracing. The only relative indications for surgery have been failure of conservative measures resulting in progressive curvature and pain. Rarely, neurologic or cardiopulmonary compromise as well as unacceptable cosmesis may lead to the invasive correction of the kyphotic deformity. The long-term outcome studies comparing conservative versus surgical treatment measures have however demonstrated no difference in the outcome of the degree of kyphosis related to the method of treatment.

Introduction

The Danish surgeon Holger Werfel Scheuermann was the first to describe the structural kyphosis of the thoracic or thoracolumbar vertebrae in 1920 [1]. The aptly named Scheuermann's disease is the most frequent cause of kyphosis in the adolescent. It is frequently misdiagnosed as postural kyphosis due to its similar presentation. The Scoliosis Research Society has defined a range from 20 and 45 degrees of thoracic kyphosis as normal for growing adolescents. Any presentation of kyphosis in the thoracolumbar junction or lumbar vertebrae is considered pathological [7].

The definitions of the deformity vary. Some physicians proposed that a global thoracic kyphosis with an angle greater than 40 degrees, irregular end plates and a minimum of one vertebra angled a minimum of 5 degrees are findings which are sufficient for a diagnosis [2]. Bradford recommended using the criterion of only one or more vertebrae wedged a minimum of 5 degrees, leading to an earlier diagnosis and consequently earlier therapeutic intervention [3]. Sorensen's radiographic criterion of the existence of at least three adjacent vertebrae angled at a minimum of 5 degrees however has been the most widely accepted amongst the medical community [4].

Sorensen originally estimated an incidence of 0.4-8.3% in 1964 [4]. This was supported by a review of 1,384 cadaveric specimens in 1991 upon which a prevalence of 7.4% was reported [5]. Despite the fact that the prevalence of Scheuermann's kyphosis is broadly considered to be equal in males and females, various studies have reported differently. Sorensen and Murray et al. reported an increased prevalence in men, with male-to-female ratios of 1.38:1 and 2.1:1, respectively [4, 6]. Bradford on the other hand reported a twice as high prevalence in female than in male individuals [7].

Scheuermann's kyphosis can be classified into three forms based on the position of the apex of the deformity. The classic thoracic form (type I) is defined by an apex localized between T7 and T9, whilst the thoracolumbar form (type II) presents with an apex localized between T10 and T12 at the thoracolumbar junction [8]. The lumbar form of the disease resulting in a loss of lumbar lordosis has been linked to athletically active male patients and can typically be resolved with activity modification and rest [9]. It has further been suggested that Scheuermann's disease of the thoracolumbar or lumbar spine is frequently overlooked or not connected to the presenting complaints of the patient by the attending physician [10].

Anatomical studies have shown lax-appearing cartilage in the vertebral end plates. Additionally, histological studies have demonstrated a dysbalance of the cartilaginous endplates' matrix components with an increase in mucopolysaccharides and a decrease in collagen. The overall organization of the collagen fibrils is poor [11]. These histological characteristics of affected end plates have been theorized to result in defective endochondral ossification, thereby stunting vertical growth [12].

The challenge that has been presented to scientists and physicians alike has been to uncover the etiology of Scheuermann's disease, to optimize existing treatment modalities, and to explore new approaches for the benefit of the patient.

Pathogenesis

Many different hypotheses have been proposed to elucidate the pathogenesis of Scheuermann's disease. Though different studies have reported a variety of data, no conclusive evidence has been found to illuminate the deformities' etiology so far. Two main divisions exist amongst the theories. The first division postulates that a change in the vertebral end plate's biochemical composition results in a loss of the biomechanical integrity of the functional spinal unit as a whole. The second division on the other hand posits that an anomaly in the patients' anatomy or motion produces abnormal mechanical stress, thereby culminating in an alteration of the biochemical composition of the endplate. Either way, the resulting focal disruption of the endochondral ossification of the end plates culminates in the osteochondrosis responsible for the kyphotic malformation of the spine.

The importance of genetics in the etiology of Scheuermann's disease remains one of the most controversially discussed topics in relation to the disease. Halal et al. reported on five families which were thought to demonstrate an autosomal dominant pattern of inheritance with a high degree of penetration but variable expression [13]. Graat et al. discussed Scheuermann's kyphosis in male monozygotic twins. Although the disease was noted on identical vertebral levels in the siblings, the Cobb angles differed greatly (74 degrees *vs.* 48 degrees) and neither of the parents showed any sign of a deformity [14]. The largest cohort study to date is based upon the Danish Twin Registry. The authors reported a heritability of 74% after evaluating a health questionnaire which included a question about Scheuermann's disease mailed to 46,418 mono- and dizygotic twins born from 1931 through 1982 [15]. However, no concrete genes have been identified so far.

It has been hypothesized that Scheuermann's kyphosis is no more than a manifestation of a generalized skeletal disease. The most prominent theory was proposed by Bradford, who noted aberrations in 12 juvenile patients' mineral parameters such as bone density, levels of serum alkaline phosphatase and urinary hydroxyproline. The author further speculated that the deformity resulted from relative osteoporosis, which manifested itself during growth spurts in adolescence [16]. A subsequent study however has found no significant difference in trabecular lumbar vertebral body bone density between adolescents diagnosed with Scheuermann's kyphosis and age-, sex-, and race-matched control subjects [17].

Mechanical factors have also been discussed as contributing elements in the deformities etiology. Scheuermann noted that children performing physical labor were more likely to develop the disease than inactive children [1]. The fact that bracing can be used to achieve pain relief and a partial correction of the kyphosis supports this theory [18]. Atypical biomechanical stresses due to physical activities or anatomic anomalies have been posited to increase compressive forces on the anterior end plates. Fotiadis et al. measured sternum length in 10,057 students. He found that the 175 patients who had been diagnosed with Scheuermann's kyphosis exhibited a shorter sternum in relationship with greater height than their healthy peers. He surmised that the shorter sternum led to a pathophysiological increase in biomechanical stress on the anterior edge of the end plate, resulting in defective growth and vertebral wedging [19]. In another study, significantly higher values for weight, height and body mass index (BMI) were found in the 175 adolescents with Scheuermann's kyphosis in comparison to the control group. No correlation however was noted between the values and the magnitude of the deformity [2]. Skogland et al. focused on the role of height, examining 62 girls for spinal deformities who had presented at his department because of above average height. He found that 18 patients exhibited kyphosis of more than 40° in the thoracic spine [20].

To date, no evidence has been found to conclusively support any of the suggested theories. In fact, Scheuermann's kyphosis appears to be a multifactorial disease.

Diagnosis

Clinical Presentation

The most frequent age of onset of Scheuermann's kyphosis is 10-12 years, but some patients may not present until adulthood [21]. Pain has been reported as a complaint in 20-60% of patients with Scheuermann's kyphosis [7]. The reasons for seeking medical attention differ in the adolescent and the adult patient population. Adolescents and their friends and family are often most concerned about the progressive kyphosis of the thoracic spine thereby causing a cosmetic anomaly. The adolescents' self-consciousness and the attribution of the kyphosis to poor posture may prevent a timely diagnosis. Adults usually present due to complications arising from the deformity, with pain being the most frequent complaint [21]. Rarely, neurologic or cardiopulmonary compromise may be the reasons for presentation. Generally, patients with a severe short-segment angular deformity are thought to be at the highest risk for these potentially life-threatening complications. Neurologic complications stemming from disk herniations, dural cysts or severe kyphosis resulting in spinal cord tethering over the apex of the deformity have been described in some patients. Disk herniations most commonly occur at the apex of the deformity due to the increased level of biomechanical stress causing more rapid degeneration [22, 23]. Cord compression secondary to the deformity may present in a variety of ways ranging from radiculopathy to paraplegia. One study reported an average of 95 degrees of kyphosis in patients presenting with neurological compromise [24]. Ryan et al. in contrast reported an average of 54 degrees of kyphosis in three patients with neurological complications secondary to their deformity [25].

Natural History

To this day, no studies discussing the natural history of patient's with Scheuermann's kyphosis who do not undergo treatment have been published in the English literature. Thorough long-term outcomes of various treatment modalities of the deformity have yet to be evaluated and reported. It has been postulated that Scheuermann's kyphosis causes greater distress in the forms of back pain and fatigue in the adolescent than in the skeletally mature adult. In the majority of cases, the deformity will not progress and will not disable the patient. Scheuermann's kyphosis type II is more likely to result in painful and progressive deformity in the adult than type I [26]. Murray et al. followed patients with a wide range of deformity (mean Scheuermann's kyphosis of 72 degrees) for an average of 32 years and found them to be generally unlimited by their disease. The study subjects were however more concerned about their appearance and worked in jobs with lower physical demands than the average population. With the progression of time, the cosmetic concerns receded. Although the prevalence of lower back pain was higher in individuals with Scheuermann's disease, the time on sick leave off work due to back pain was equal to that of individuals without the disease. Exclusively patients with a kyphosis of more than 85 degrees were more often single than their age- and gender-matched control subjects. These patients were also noted to have a lower inspiratory capacity. Overall, no significant differences were recorded for the Scheuermann's kyphosis patient's level of education, recreational activities, perceived physical activity level or need for pain medication [6].

Physical Examination

Scheuermann's kyphosis is characterized by rigid structural thoracic or thoracolumbar hyperkyphosis which is typically accompanied by several additional morphological features. The excessive kyphosis may result in pelvic anteversion, shoulder rounding and lumbar as well as cervical hyperlordosis. The shortened trunk results in relatively long appearing arms and legs. When viewed from the side, the apex of the curve and the overall kyphosis can be easily delineated. Depending on the level of compensatory lumbar hyperlordosis, sagittal balance may or may not be maintained. The deformity may retain a small element of correction upon hyperextension and flexion, but will generally remain rigid. Localized tenderness around the apex of the kyphosis is a common finding. Muscular tension, particularly of the hamstring and the iliopsoas, will frequently contribute to pain experienced by the patient. Additional back pain due to a variety of causes such as concomitant degenerative disk disease, spondylosis or cysts may be identified upon palpation. Approximately one third of the individuals presenting with Scheuermann's disease have concomitant spondylolysis of L5, spondylolisthesis or mild scoliosis and will consequently exhibit additional symptoms caused by these diseases [27]. A thorough neurological examination should identify any sensory or motor deficits, which may have resulted from the disease. In patients with severe deformity, a cardiopulmonary examination to rule out any spatial compromise may be warranted.

Differential Diagnosis

The most prominent differential diagnosis of Scheuermann's kyphosis is postural round-back kyphosis. The presentation may mimic that of milder cases of Scheuermann's kyphosis quite closely, but the diseases can be differentiated based on a few key findings. Postural kyphosis generally does not have a curve of more than 60 degrees.

The deformity will appear smooth and never short-segmented, with a clearly delineated apex. Although postural hyperkyphosis may become somewhat rigid with age, it is usually correctable in hyperextension. Finally, the vertebrae will not exhibit any of the findings typical for Scheuermann's kyphosis. The motion segments involved in the kyphosis will not appear to be out of order, with age appropriate signs of disk degeneration, no vertebral wedging and no irregularities of the endplates.

Imaging

To allow for adequate primary evaluation, standard postero-anterior (PA) and lateral full-spine standing radiographs should be obtained for all patients. At least three adjacent wedged vertebrae angled at a minimum of 5 degrees are the defining finding for most physicians when establishing the diagnosis of Scheuermann's kyphosis, as demonstrated in Figure 1 in a 13 year old female with 73 degrees of kyphosis and back pain [4]. The apex and the expanse of the deformity should be defined. The lateral film allows for the evaluation of spino-pelvic parameters and sagittal balance. The degree of kyphosis should be captured from the most distal to the most proximal vertebrae included in the deformity using the Cobb method [6]. The PA films may demonstrate concomitant scoliosis. Edgren's sign, a compensational lengthening of vertebrae's adjacent to a flattened vertebral body, may also be observed. Attempts have been made to identify new radiographic characteristics of the onset of Scheuermann's disease to allow for an earlier diagnosis and subsequent earlier initiation of treatment. Mallet et al. for example identified a projection of the ring apophysis underneath the endplate, which appeared before the onset of vertebral wedging [28]. If patients are considered for surgical treatment, a magnetic resonance imaging (MRI) of the spine as well as a supine hyperextension lateral radiograph should be obtained. The supine hyperextension (over a bolster) lateral radiograph allows for the determination of the structural degree of the deformity. The MRI on the other hand allows for a closer evaluation of the disk impairment and endplate irregularities, and may identify cysts, stenosis and other potential causes of neurological complications.

Management

The majority of Scheuermann's kyphosis patients are treated non-operatively. No long-term studies have evaluated the efficacy of one treatment over another. Treatment options for Scheuermann's kyphosis include, but are not limited to, lifestyle modification and observation, physical therapy, pain management, bracing and surgery. The treatment modality selected for Scheuermann's kyphosis patients should be based on the degree of severity and the apex of the kyphosis, the pain severity and the degree of dissatisfaction of the patients with their appearance. The opinions on the correct utilization of bracing or surgery as treatment measures for the adolescent *vs.* the adult are divergent.

Conservative Management

Observation

In patients with mild curves, whose kyphosis is <55 degrees in the thoracic spine for Scheuermann's kyphosis type I or <40 degrees for Scheuermann's kyphosis type II, initial observation and life style modifications may be warranted [26]. Since the disease has a generally benign course, patients who do not experience further complaints may not require any further treatment. Physical activity placing pressure on the vertebrae, such as weight lifting for recreational or professional purposes, and with repetitive strains to the spine, such as contact sports, should be avoided. The development of the patient's spine curvature and symptom evolution should be monitored closely. Progressive deformity or the onset of pain in patients may warrant the initiation of active additional conservative or surgical management.

Pain Medication

Nonsteroidal anti-inflammatory drugs can be a useful approach in the treatment for lower back pain secondary to spondylosis, neurological complications or herniated disks stemming from the premature disk degeneration. They may also be used as a short-term supplement to conservative management of the skeletally immature patient.

Physical Therapy

The goal of physical therapy is not so much to lessen the kyphosis than to improve general physical conditioning and alleviate pain [29]. The exercises are designed to alleviate muscular tension secondary to the deformity and include hamstrings stretching, postural improvement exercises and trunk extensor strengthening. Back pain secondary to spondylosis in the adult patient may benefit from core spinal stabilization exercises. Physical therapy is primarily recommended for patients experiencing pain with mild or slightly correctible deformity or as a supplement to bracing to prevent stiffening. A study followed 351 patients between 17 and 21 years of age with Scheuermann's kyphosis who presented with pain and underwent a program consisting of exercise, manual therapy, and osteopathy for pain management.

It reported a 16-32% reduction in pain and decreased frequency of pain in the patients [30].

Bracing

Bracing aims to slow the progression of the deformity and achieve partial curve correction by reducing the strain on the vertebral endplates. It may thereby relieve pain. Bracing is generally indicated for symptomatic Scheuermann's kyphosis adolescent patients with a mild curve ranging from 45-65 degrees. A study looking at the effects of brace treatment in adults however did find significant improvement despite the skeletal maturity of the patients. Bradford et al. evaluated 75 patients who received brace treatment for an average of 34.3 months, and reported an average of a 40% improvement of the kyphosis after a mean follow up of 14.3 months [31]. Despite this success rate, bracing is generally poorly tolerated due to the aesthetic and psychological impacts on the individual and therefore usually plays a limited role for the adult patient. Long-term follow-up was not available for the patients. The brace most commonly utilized for classic Scheuermann's kyphosis type I is the Milwaukee brace, which extends from the pelvis to the anterior cranial aspect of the sternum. The brace spans the entire torso, with a posterior sacral support and a high anterior support. A smaller brace, the underarm brace, consists of a more limited posterior support at the apex of the deformity and two anterior supports that counterbalance the first. It is indicated for both the thoracic type I as well the thoracolumbar type II pattern of kyphosis. Bracing treatment benefits from an early initiation of treatment. In the treatment of the adolescent, it should be worn 21 hours per day until the patient reaches skeletal maturity and the deformity has stabilized [29]. Sachs et al. followed 120 patients who had completed Milwaukee brace treatment for a minimum of 5 years after the completion of treatment. The average age at the patient's last follow-up examination was 24 years, with an average age of 12.4 at the initiation of treatment. Of the compliant patients, 66% showed a 10-20% improvement of the initial kyphosis and 24% showed a worsening. A total of 10% of the patients presented with a degree of kyphosis similar to the kyphosis before bracing [32]. A plaster cast may be indicated for 1–3 months for severely rigid kyphosis, with unsatisfactory compliance or for treatment of the adolescent bordering skeletal maturity. In general, bracing may also be used to alleviate severe pain as well as neurologic or cardiopulmonary compromise in patients who are contraindicated for surgical treatment.

Surgical Management

Progression of the kyphosis, pain associated with the deformity, neurologic or cardiopulmonary compromise, and cosmesis may all be indications for surgical intervention. Surgery should ideally be performed on skeletally mature patients after other conservative management measures have failed. The goal of surgical management of Scheuermann's kyphosis is to correct the degree of curvature of the kyphosis and maintain that correction through solid fusion. Patients with a painful rigid kyphosis of more than 80 degrees in the thoracic spine or of more than 65 degrees in the thoracolumbar spine resisting correction or pain relief during bracing and other conservative management measures or patients with sagittal imbalance secondary to their deformity may be indicated for surgery. Patients with severe curves who suffer from neurologic or cardiopulmonary complications secondary to the deformity should be operated on emergently to halt a deterioration of the general health of the individual [26, 33, 34]. Due to the invasive nature of the surgery, intraoperative neuromonitoring of somatosensory and motor-evoked potentials should be performed. The entire length of the kyphosis should be fused. Lowe and Kasten recommended including the first lordotic segment distal of the deformity into the instrumented fusion to avoid the development of adjacent segment disease. Additionally, they recommended to correct no more than 50% of the degree of original curve to avoid junctional kyphosis [35].

Anterior-Only Approach

The anterior-only approach described by Kostuik is an anterior interbody release and fusion with the implementation of a Harrington rod distraction system. The surgery is designed to be followed by a period of post-operative bracing. Advantages include an adequate anterior release and the establishment of an arthrodesis under compression forces. In a study of 36 skeletally mature patients diagnosed with Scheuermann's kyphosis, he reported a reduction of deformity from a mean of 75.5 degrees of preoperative curvature to a mean of 60 degrees postoperatively [36]. Despite this, the anterior-only surgical technique is not widely used.

Posterior-Only Approach

The posterior-only approach is generally recommended to patients with a flexible deformity that mildly corrects on hyperextension radiographs to <50 degrees [18]. Patients with a rigid or particularly severe curve as well as patients with anterior bridging osteophytes may be contra-indicated for this procedure [37]. The posterior-only approach was the first surgical technique described to manage Scheuermann's kyphosis [38]. In a study published in 1975, poorer results in terms of loss of correction of the curvature were found with posterior-only approach in comparison with combined anterior-posterior approach [39]. No release of the anterior longitudinal ligament can take place during a posterior-only procedure, resulting in a persistent tensile strain placed on the instrumentation. This may have led to the higher rates of hardware failure and pseudoarthrosis which were initially captured for this approach in the study compared with procedures that included an anterior release. With the development of new technologies, the introduction of dual rods and the advent of multiple segmental fixation for optimal bone purchase, posterior instrumentation can now resist the strain of the anterior longitudinal ligament and open up the intervertebral disk spaces [37]. Novel surgical techniques such as pedicle screw fixation and Ponte osteotomies have continued the improvement of the results for posterior-only approach arthrodesis [30]. A posterior only approach with four-level Ponte osteotomies around the apex of the deformity are demonstrated in Figure 2. The 13-year old female received a posterior spinal fusion from T2 to the first lordotic vertebra at L3 which corrected her kyphosis from 78 degrees to 43 degrees.

Combined Anterior-Posterior Approach

The combined anterior-posterior approach is recommended for patients with severe, rigid kyphosis of more than 75 degrees, which does not correct with hyperextension as well as patients with evidence of anterior osteophyte bridging [18]. The anterior and the posterior approach can be performed on the same setting or at different stages, depending on the disposition of the patient. The anterior approach, which may be performed through an open approach or thoracoscopically, allows for the anterior release of spine structures. The posterior approach subsequently allows for the correction of the kyphosis and the instrumented fusion. Herrera-Soto et al. [41] described 19 patients who underwent surgery using the combined antero-posterior approach with a thoracoscopic anterior release (video-assisted thoracoscopic surgery). A mean pre-operative curvature of 84.8 degrees was corrected to a mean of 45.3 degrees with a minimal mean loss of 1.6 degrees of correction at follow-up. Despite using a minimally invasive technique for the anterior approach however, 26% of the patients developed pulmonary complications.

Complications

Encouraging results have been reported for the surgical management of Scheuermann's kyphosis in terms of correction of the deformity and alleviating pain. The inherent risks of such extensive surgery however must be carefully evaluated individually for each patient. The most frequent complications associated with the surgical treatment of Scheuermann's kyphosis are neurological deficits, infection, and pulmonary compromise [42]. Additionally, junctional kyphosis requiring revision surgery to include the afflicted adjacent vertebra in the fusion construct has been described extensively in the literature [43]. The posterior-only approach has the advantage of being associated with a decreased blood loss and avoiding delicate vascular and visceral structures susceptible to injury during an anterior approach.

Outcomes

Soo et al. evaluated 63 patients with Scheuermann's kyphosis at a mean follow-up of 14 years after the completion of treatment. Patients received either an exercise regimen with observation, Milwaukee bracing or fusion with the Harrington system. The authors found that there were no differences in the patient's social or academic status, general health, career, or degree of pain between Scheuermann's kyphosis type I and type II, the treatment modality and the degree of the curvature [44].

Conclusion

Scheuermann's disease is defined by the wedging of at least three adjacent vertebral bodies angled a minimum of 5 degrees. The degree of the curve as well as the symptoms and disability caused by the disease vary widely amongst patients. The unclear etiology of Scheuermann's kyphosis makes treatment a challenge. Nonetheless, a careful selection of the appropriate treatment regimen for each patient based on the individual's age, bone status, back pain, degree of kyphosis and potential neurological or cardiopulmonary complications allows for excellent treatment results.

References

[1] Scheuermann H. Kyfosis dorsalis juvenilis. *Ugeskr Laeger* [in Danish]. 1920; 82:385–93.

[2] Fotiadis E, Kenanidis E, Samoladas E et al. Scheuermann's disease: focus on weight and height role. *Eur Spine J.* 2008 May; 17(5):673-8.

[3] Holt RT, Dopf CA, Isaza JE, et al. Adult kyphosis. In: Frymoyer JW, ed. *The Adult Spine. Principles and Practice.* 2nd ed. Philadelphia, PA: Lippincott Williams & Wilkins. 1997:1537-1578.

[4] Sorensen K. *Scheuermann's juvenile kyphosis.* Copenhague: Munskgaard; 1964.

[5] Scoles PV, Latimer BM, DigIovanni BF et al. Vertebral alterations in Scheuermann's kyphosis. *Spine.* 1991 May; 16(5):509-15.

[6] Murray PM, Weinstein SL, Spratt KF. The natural history and long-term follow-up of Scheuermann kyphosis. *J Bone Joint Surg Am.* 1993 Feb; 75(2):236-48.

[7] Bradford DS. Juvenile Kyphosis, in Bradford DS, Lonstein JE, Moe JH, Ogilvie JW, Winter RB (eds): *Moe's Textbook of Scoliosis and other Spinal Deformities,* 2nd ed. WB Saunders. 1987: pp 347-368.

[8] Wood KB, Melikian R, Villamil F. Adult Scheuermann kyphosis: evaluation, management, and new developments. *J Am Acad Orthop Surg.* 2012 Feb; 20(2):113-21.

[9] Wenger D, Frick S. Scheuermann kyphosis. *Spine.* 1999; 24(24):2630-2369.

[10] Lings S, Mikkelsen L. Scheuermann's disease with low localization. A problem of under-diagnosis. *Scand J Rehabil Med.* 1982; 14(2):77-9.

[11] Ippolito E, Bellocci M, Montanaro A et al. Juvenile kyphosis: an ultrastructural study. *J Pediatr Orthop.* 1985 May-Jun; 5(3):315-22.

[12] Aufdermaur M. Juvenile kyphosis (Scheuermann's disease): radiography, histology, and pathogenesis. *Clin Orthop Relat Res.* 1981 Jan-Feb; (154):166-74.

[13] Halal F, Gledhill RB, Fraser C. Dominant inheritance of Scheuermann's juvenile kyphosis. *Am J Dis Child.* 1978 Nov; 132(11):1105-7.

[14] Graat H1, van Rhijn LW, Schrander-Stumpel CT et al. Classical Scheuermann disease in male monozygotic twins: further support for the genetic etiology hypothesis. *Spine.* 2002 Nov 15; 27(22):E485-7.

[15] Damborg F, Engell V, Andersen M. Genetic epidemiology of Scheuermann's disease. *Acta Orthop.* 2011 Oct; 82(5):602-5.

[16] Bradford DS, Brown DM, Moe JH. Scheuermann's kyphosis: a form of osteoporosis? *Clin Orthop Relat Res*. 1976 Jul-Aug; (118):10-5.

[17] Gilsanz V, Gibbens DT, Carlson M. Vertebral bone density in Scheuermann disease. *J Bone Joint Surg Am*. 1989 Jul; 71(6):894-7.

[18] Tribus CB. Scheuermann's kyphosis in adolescents and adults: diagnosis and management. *J Am Acad Orthop Surg*. 1998 Jan-Feb; 6(1):36-43.

[19] Fotiadis E, Grigoriadou A, Kapetanos G. The role of sternum in the etiopathogenesis of Scheuermann disease of the thoracic spine. *Spine*. 2008 Jan 1; 33(1):E21-4.

[20] Skogland LB, Steen H, Trygstad O. Spinal deformities in tall girls. *Acta Orthop Scand*. 1985 Apr; 56(2):155-7.

[21] Wood KB, Melikian R, Villamil F. Adult Scheuermann kyphosis: evaluation, management, and new developments. *J Am Acad Orthop Surg*. 2012 Feb; 20(2):113-21.

[22] Yablon JS, Kasdon DL, Levine H. Thoracic cord compression in Scheuermann's disease. *Spine* (Phila Pa 1976). 1988 Aug; 13(8):896-8.

[23] Chiu KY, Luk KD. Cord compression caused by multiple disc herniations and intraspinal cyst in Scheuermann's disease. *Spine* (Phila Pa 1976). 1995 May 1; 20(9):1075-9.

[24] Lonstein JE, Winter RB, Moe JH. Neurologic deficits secondary to spinal deformity. A review of the literature and report of 43 cases. *Spine* (Phila Pa 1976). 1980 Jul-Aug; 5(4):331-55.

[25] Ryan MD, Taylor TK. Acute spinal cord compression in Scheuermann's disease. *J Bone Joint Surg Br*. 1982; 64(4):409-12.

[26] Lowe TG. Scheuermann disease. *J Bone Joint Surg Am*. 1990 Jul; 72(6):940-5.

[27] Ali RM, Green DW, Patel TC. Scheuermann's kyphosis. *Curr Opin Pediatr*. 1999 Feb; 11(1):70-5.

[28] Mallet J, Rey JC, Raimbeau G, Senly G. [Scheuermann's disease. Spinal growth dystrophy]. *Rev Prat*. 1984 Jan 1; 34(1):29-39.

[29] Zaina F, Atanasio S, Ferraro C, et al. Review of rehabilitation and orthopedic conservative approach to sagittal plane diseases during growth: Hyperkyphosis, junctional kyphosis, and Scheuermann disease. *Eur J Phys Rehabil Med* 2009; 45(4):595-603.

[30] Weiss HR, Dieckmann J, Gerner HJ. Effect of intensive rehabilitation on pain in patients with Scheuermann's disease. *Stud Health Technol Inform* 2002; 88: 254-257.

[31] Bradford DS, Moe JH, Montalvo FJ et al. Scheuermann's kyphosis and roundback deformity: Results of Milwaukee brace treatment. *J Bone Joint Surg Am* 1974; 56(4):740-758.

[32] Sachs B, Bradford D, Winter R, et al. Scheuermann kyphosis. Follow-up of Milwaukee brace treatment. *J Bone Joint Surg Am* 1987; 69:50–7.

[33] Lowe TG. Scheuermann's disease. In: DeWald RL, editor. *Textbook of spine surgery*. Philadelphia: Lippincott- Raven; 1997. p. 1173–98.

[34] Bradford DS, Ahmed KB, Moe JH, et al. The surgical management of patients with Scheuermann's disease. *J Bone Joint Surg Am* 1980; 62:705–12.

[35] Lowe TG, Kasten MD. An analysis of sagittal curves and balance after Cotrel- Dubousset instrumentation for kyphosis secondary to Scheuermann's disease: A review of 32 patients. *Spine* (Phila Pa 1976) 1994; 19(15):1680-1685.

[36] Kostuik JP. Anterior Kostuik-Harrington distraction systems. *Orthopedics* 1988; 11(10):1379-1391.

[37] Sturm PF, Dobson JC, Armstrong GW. The surgical management of Scheuermann's disease. *Spine* (Phila Pa 1976) 1993; 18(6):685-691.

[38] Papagelopoulos PJ, Mavrogenis AF, Savvidou OD, et al. Current concepts in Scheuermann's kyphosis. *Orthopedics* 2008; 31:52–8, quiz 9–60.

[39] Bradford DS, Moe JH, Montalvo FJ et al. Scheuermann's kyphosis: Results of surgical treatment by posterior spine arthrodesis in twenty-two patients. *J Bone Joint Surg Am* 1975; 57(4):439- 448.

[40] Geck MJ, Macagno A, Ponte A, et al. The Ponte procedure: Posterior only treatment of Scheuermann's kyphosis using segmental posterior shortening and pedicle screw instrumentation. *J Spinal Disord Tech* 2007; 20(8):586-593.

[41] Herrera-Soto JA, Parikh SN, Al-Sayyad MJ, et al. Experience with combined video-assisted thoracoscopic surgery (VATS) anterior spinal release and posterior spinal fusion in Scheuermann's kyphosis. *Spine* 2005; 30:2176-81.

[42] Lowe TG, Line BG. Evidence based medicine: analysis of Scheuermann kyphosis. *Spine* (Phila Pa 1976) 2007; 32:S115–9.

[43] Kim HJ, Lenke LG, Shaffrey CI, et al. Proximal junctional kyphosis as a distinct form of adjacent segment pathology after spinal deformity surgery: a systematic review. *Spine* (Phila Pa 1976) 2012; 37:S144–64.

[44] C.L. Soo, MD, Philip C. Noble, PhD, Stephen I. Esses, MD. Scheuermann kyphosis: long-term follow-up. *Spine J.* 2002 Jan-Feb; 2(1):49-56.

In: Kyphosis
Editor: Janice Newton

ISBN: 978-1-63483-224-3

Chapter V

Intraocular Surgery in Kyphosis

Mohannad Qasim Albdour*[1], *MD,
and Karanjit S. Kooner*[*,2], *MD, PhD
[1,2] Department of Ophthalmology,
University of Texas Southwestern medical Center, Dallas, TX, US
[2] Currently at Department of Ophthalmology,
King Hussein Medical Center, Amman, Jordan

Abstract

Kyphosis is a progressive, curvature of thoracic spine which results in rounding or bowing of the back . Curved spine accompanied by restricted neck motion and poor lung reserve present challenges for an ophthalmic surgeon who is used to patient's neck and head resting flat on the operating table and the eye in the horizontal position. Intraoperative difficulties include poor view, inability to maneuver surgical instruments properly and constant threat of elevated vitreous pressure. Several innovative solutions have been published including, maximal reverse Trendelenburg position with pillows under the head and neck, use of a donut and wedge shaped head positioner, allowing the patient to remain

[*] Correspondence address: Karanjit S. Kooner, MD PhD, Associate Professor, Department of Ophthalmology, University of Texas Southwestern Medical Center; 5323 Harry Hines Blvd.; Dallas, Texas 75390-9057. Tel No: 214/648-4733. ax No: 214/648-2270. Email: Karanjit.Kooner@UTSouthwestern.edu.

in upright sitting position while their head is positioned horizontally in a modified waiting room chair, performing surgery while standing, using 4-section orthopedic operating table, laying the patients on their sides, *side saddle* positioning, face-to-face positioning, parachute type harness inferior corneal retraction suture, or extreme patient positioning for retinal surgery. This chapter highlights various surgical options to facilitate surgeons pick the best course of action when dealing with intraocular surgery in patients with kyphosis.

Keywords: intraocular surgery, kyphosis

Introduction

Intraocular microsurgery mandates comfortable seating of both the patient and the surgeon at the start of the surgery. If either of these pre requisites is compromised, the ensuing suboptimal view of the eye may result in a high chance of intraocular complications. Patients with kyphosis present multitude of challenges related to their physical disabilities including concomitant pulmonary and cardiovascular diseases [1]. Several practical solutions have been described by very experienced surgeons but complications may still occur [2].

Gordon et al. were able to successfully complete cataract surgery on a patient with severe kyphosis by using three pillows under his head and neck and 11 pillows under patient's buttocks and legs with the operating table positioned in maximum reverse Trendelenburg position [3]. They stressed that pillows be securely taped to the operating table to prevent slippage. A wedge-shaped pillow with built-in donut for positioning of the head and back [Profex Medical Products, St. Louis, MO] has been used by some surgeons [4]. This allows patient's head to be extended forward thus making the eye more accessible for surgery. They recommended using more than one of these positioners in severe cases. The depth of the doughnut helps to fix as well as elevate the head.

Fine and associates modified a common waiting room chair, for less than $ 200, to accommodate patients with various back and head disabilities and enable these patients to remain in an upright seated position and tilt their head back [5]. The back cushion of the chair was placed on adjustable brackets. The legs of the chair were shortened to allow the patients to stretch their legs out in front to counterbalance the tilted position of the back and head. An adjustable head rest clamp was attached to the back of the chair to provide firm support. Extra stability was provided by a spindle attached to a strut between the front legs of the chair for counterbalance. Authors felt that their patients did not experience the cognitive and anoxia related symptoms in a supine position.

Another approach suggested performing cataract surgery standing up using loupes for magnification and fiber optic headlamp for coaxial illumination and making an infero-temporal scleral tunnel [6]. This surgery was complicated by posterior capsular tear requiring anterior vitrectomy. The surgeons were also unable to remove sub-incisional cortex because of shallow anterior chamber secondary to elevated posterior vitreous pressure. Poor visualization and unaccustomed standing position may have contributed to the complications. Hunter was able to remove cataract in an obese patient by performing phacoemulsification while standing but needed an ophthalmic technician to control focusing and side movements of the microscope [7]. A national survey of ophthalmic surgeons in United Kingdom reported that over 50% did perform cataract surgery while standing, if required [8]. A prospective study in England also showed that standing phacoemulsification was as safe as conventional surgery in the hands of experienced surgeons provided patient specific measures were taken [9].

Prasad et al. recommended using a 4-section orthopedic operating table to enable an extreme reverse Trendelenburg position for cataract and glaucoma surgery [10]. However, because of blurred vision, they were unable to perform curvilinear capsulorehexis and had to resort to can-opener capsulotomy. Sambandam was able to complete cataract surgery on a patient with severe kyphosis by laying her on her side [11]. This patient was unable to lie on her back at all. A side saddle approach was described by Nair et al. where in the surgeon sat with his thighs parallel to the long axis of the operating table and facing the head end [12]. The optical axis of the microscope had to be inclined about 60° towards the horizontal. The globe was tilted superotemporally to optimize red reflex. They used intra cameral anesthesia and infero-temporal corneal incision which may increase incidence of endophthalmitis. When the patient can only be placed in a semi recumbent position, Ang et al. have proposed a face-to-face sitting position and tilting the operating microscope 60° from the vertical [13]. Surgeon has to be aware and adjust for the unsteadiness caused by outstretched arms. Topical anesthesia allowed the patient to comply with requests to fixate on the microscope light. Some patients may need strong parachute-like support harness for secure positioning [14]. The surgeons used foam to support the head, neck, shoulders and knees and moved the table in extreme Trendelenburg position. They used Velcro surgical straps similar to straps in a parachute harness. Cataract was removed via a superotemporal corneal approach under retrobulbar anesthesia. Elevated legs may distend jugular veins and result in increased posterior pressure.

We described a 49- year-old obese male with controlled secondary glaucoma who needed cataract surgery in the right eye [15]. He had ankylosing spondylitis related extreme kyphosis and neck in fixed flexion (Figure 1). His pulmonary reserve was also very low. The past ocular history was positive for recurrent uveitis and glaucoma shunt surgery in the right eye. The pupil was small and fixed from posterior synechia. The cataract was +4 dense. The best corrected visual acuity was 20/200. The anterior chamber was shallow and glaucoma tube shunt was visible at 11 o'clock position. The pre-op plan included pupillary dilation with iris retraction hooks, corneal staining with trypan blue, and phacoemulsification with intra ocular implantation under local anesthesia. The anesthesiologist was reluctant to use general anesthesia because of patient's disability and poor health.

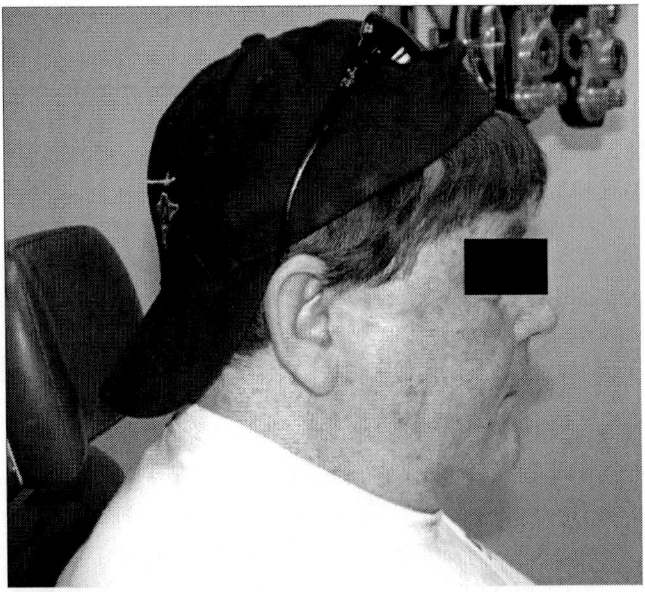

Figure 1. The patient with kyphosis and immobile neck in fixed flexion.

In the operating room, the patient could only recline to about 40° from the vertical axis despite maximal reverse Trendelenburg position and number of pillows under his back, neck, head and legs (Figure 2). With the surgeon at the temporal side of the patient, the eye was also seen reclining at 40° (Figure 3). While trying to focus the microscope, it became evident that by grasping the eye at the inferior limbus with a fine forceps, and pulling it upwards, the eye could be moved to a more desirable horizontal position. A single 7/0 Vicryl (polyglactin) corneal retraction suture was placed at the limbus at 6 o'clock position to achieve the desired view (Figure 4). The assistant was able to rotate the eye to the desired positions during the whole procedure by relaxing or pulling on the suture (Figure 5). There were no intra-ocular complications and the post-operative recovery was uneventful. The final best corrected visual acuity was 20/30.

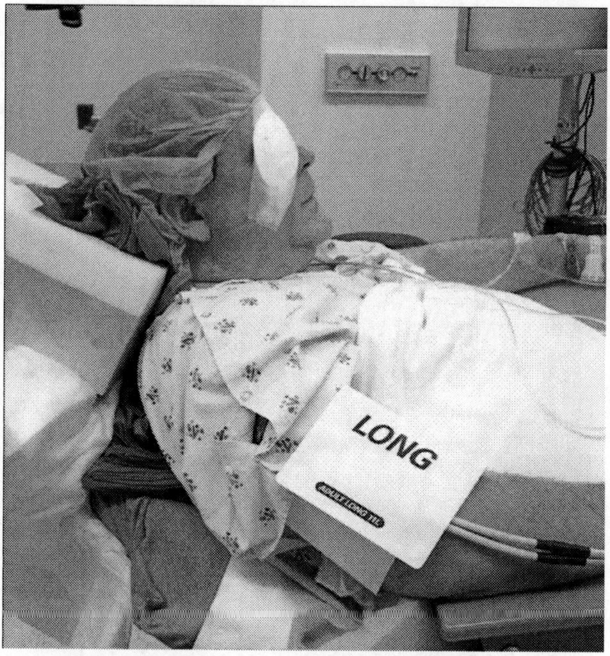

Figure 2. The position best tolerated by the patient during surgery.

Retinal surgeries are often more complex and require longer duration than cataract surgeries. You and associates [16] employed the head-down position with cushioning support in a man with severe 90 ° curvature of his spine. They used three large orthopedic cushions and several pillows to raise the patient's legs by approximately 48 ° and secured the patient with ample surgical tape and three straps. The operating microscope had to be tilted at 15 ° offset. The team was able to complete the very complex retinal procedure without any complications.

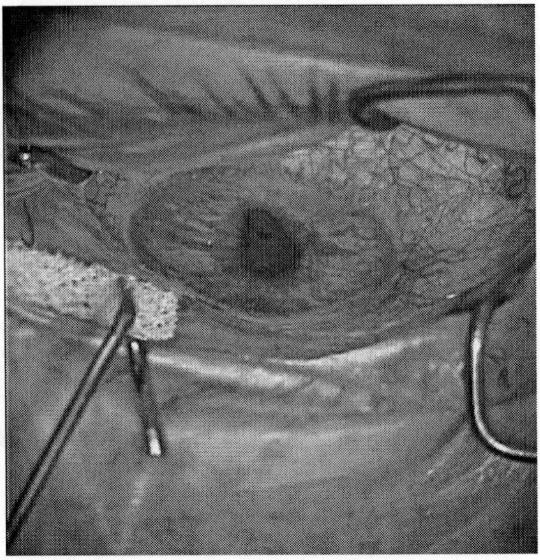

Figure 3. The virtual vertical position of the eye at the beginning of surgery.

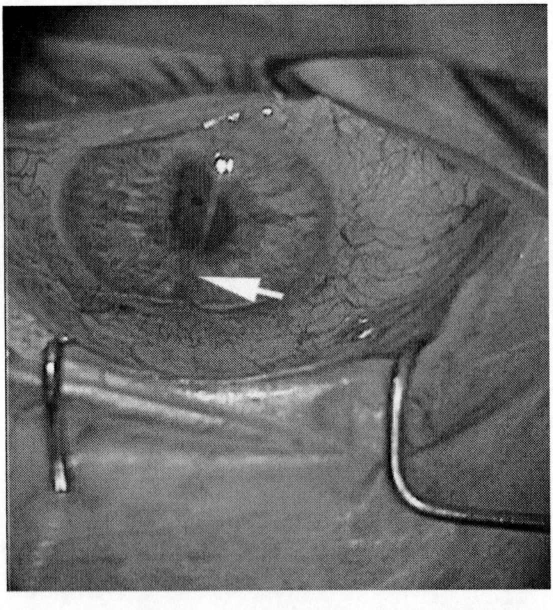

Figure 4. Pull on the corneal retraction suture (white arrow) allowed rotation of the eye more horizontally.

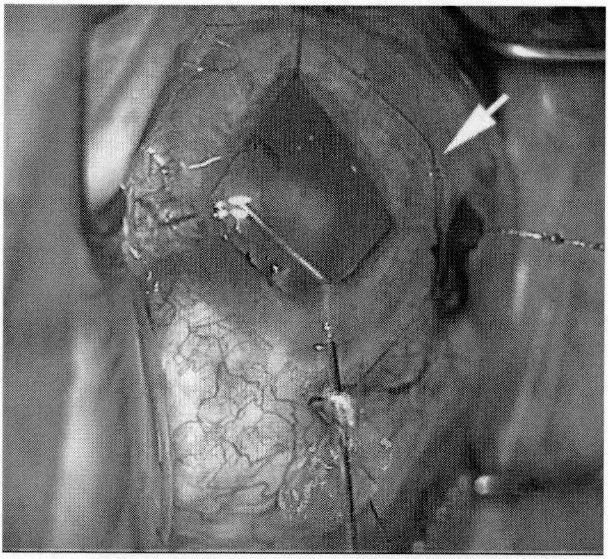

Figure 5. Cataract surgery was completed successfully. Iris retraction sutures kept the pupil dilated.

In a patient with severe thoracic kyphosis who was unable to lie flat on a table, Razeghinejad et al. used a chair with adjustable top between an operating table and another small table [17]. The wheels of the table and the chair were secured with adhesive tape. The patient was laid with his head on the small table and his thorax fitting on the well-padded chair. The adjustable top of the chair allowed accommodating kyphotic thorax. The cataract surgery was performed successfully. Packer recommended making an extra paracentesis inferiorly to assist in capsulorrhexis but the relatively vertical position of the eye still made this procedure difficult [18].

Conclusion

Patients with kyphosis may present several unique challenges to an eye surgeon. The foremost being the inability to lay the head and neck in the ideal horizontal position. The resulting poor view makes focusing and manipulation of tissues and instruments difficult. Tilting the head end of the operating table down and raising patient's legs may compromise venous return from the orbit causing venous engorgement and elevated posterior vitreous pressure during surgery. In addition, patient's poor pulmonary reserve itself may further impede orbital/jugular venous return resulting in increased posterior vitreous pressure [14, 5, 6, 9]. Afshar et al. have proposed an in-office trial of Trendelenburg positioning by inclining an office examination chair to determine head position while supine [19]. Other features of kyphosis that may adversely affect intra ocular surgery are tenderness and stiffness of the back and difficulty breathing. It is imperative that the anesthesiology and nursing staff be alerted and consulted for team work. Most experts have recommended topical, intracameral anesthesia rather than general anesthesia in patients with kyphosis [12, 19, 20]. Topical anesthesia allows the patient to fixate on the operating light, keep the eye in the desired position and obtain the best red reflex. Other helpful maneuvers are, turning the patient's face and /or chin up, standing temporal approach and using straight instruments rather than curved to avoid damaging intraocular structures [20]. In short, there is no single solution for these groups of difficult patients. Careful pre-op evaluation, planning and a team approach with internist, anesthesiologist, nursing staff is paramount. A surgeon may use one or more proven ways to deal with the issues at hand. Besides kyphosis these suggestions may also be helpful in other conditions causing inability to recline such as torticollis [21], chronic obstructive pulmonary disease, chronic congestive heart failure, morbid obesity, myotonic dystrophy, ankylosing spondylitis, cerebral palsy, Meniere's disease or claustrophobia. Surgeons may consider operating on these patients earlier when the cataract is softer rather than later to avoid complications associated with advanced hard cataracts.

Acknowledgments

Supported in part by unrestricted grant from the Society to Prevent Blindness New York, and Visual Science Core Grant EY 020799.

Authors have no financial or proprietary interest in the materials described in the article.

References

[1] Freeman BL III. Scoliosis and kyphosis. In: Canale ST, Beaty JH, eds. *Campbell's Operative Orthopaedics*. 11th ed. Philadelphia, Pa: *Mosby Elsevier;* 2007: chap 38.

[2] Rogers GM and Goins KM. Cataract surgery in the patient that cannot lie flat. *Curr Opin Ophthalmol.* 2010; 21:71-74.

[3] Gordon ML, Rodriguez AA, Olson MD, Miller KM. Pillow case. *J Cataract Refract Surg* 2005; 31: 1824-1825.

[4] Livingston M and Mackool RJ. Donut wedge cataract positioner (letter). *J Cataract Refract Surg.* 1995; 21:5-6.

[5] Fine IH, Hoffman RS, Binstock S. Phacoemulsification performed in a modified waiting room chair. *J Cataract Refract Surg.* 1996; 22:1408-1410.

[6] Rimmer S and Miller KM. Phacoemulsification in the standing position with loupe magnification and headlamp illumination. *J Cataract Refract Surg.* 1994; 20:353-354.

[7] Hunter LH. Standing while performing phacoemulsification. *J Cataract Refract Surg.* 1995; 21:111.

[8] Chandradeva K, Hugkulstone CE. Standing phacoemulsification: a national survey. *Journal of Cataract and Refractive Surgery* 2007; 32(12):2155-6. DOI:10.1016/j.jcrs.2006.06.038.

[9] Hugkulstone CE. Standing phacoemulsification: A prospective audit of 20 consecutive cases. *Journal of Cataract and Refractive Surgery* 2010; 36(10):1763-7. DOI: 10.1016/j.jcrs.2010.04.031

[10] Prasad SP, Kamath GG and Philips RP. Phacoemulsification in a patient with marked cervical kyphosis. *J Cataract Refract Surg* 2000; 26: 1258-1260.98.

[11] Sambandam SPT. Cataract extraction in a humpback woman. Indian J Ophthalmol. 1974; 22:35, available from: http://www.ijo.in/text.asp?1974/22/1/35/31381. .

[12] Nair J and Rimmer T. Side saddle cataract surgery for patients unable to lie flat: learning from the past. *Eye* 2007; 21:1122-1123. DOI:10.1038/sj.eye.6702891.

[13] Ang GS, Ong JM, Eke T. Face-to-face seated positioning for phacoemulsification in patients unable to lie flat for cataract surgery. *Am J Ophthalmol. 2006*; 141(6):1151-2.

[14] Muthialu A, Rauen M, Newsom TH, Jensen L, Oetting TA. Parachute-like harness to position patients with severe kyphosis during cataract surgery. *J Cataract Refract Surg.* 2009; 35(8):1332-4. DOI: 10.1016/j.jcrs.2009.03.027.

[15] Kooner KS and Barte FM: Intraocular surgery in kyphosis: an easier approach. *Case Rep Ophthalmol* 2013; 4:34-38. DOI: 10.1159/000353227.

[16] You T, Huang CX, Chen S, Maggiano J, Rathod R, Chang E and Casiano M. Case report: extreme patient positioning for retinal surgery in advanced kyphosis. *Retin cases Brief Rep.* 2015 (Epub ahead of print).

[17] Razeghinejad M and Eghbal M. A simple way to achieve the routine position for phacoemulsification in a patient with marked thoracic kyphosis. *J Ophthalmic Vis Res* 2009; 4 (4): 253-255.

[18] Packer M. Cataract surgery in severely kyphotic patient. Video available at http://www.surgytec.com/video/cataract-surgerykyphotic-patient.

[19] Afshar AR, Pongsachareonnont P, Siegner SW, Stewart JM. Trendelenburg positioning with temporal approach for vitreoretinal surgery in a patient with severe kyphosis. *Eye* (2014) 28, 1261–1263; doi:10.1038/eye.2014.17.

[20] Eke T. Side-saddle cataract surgery for patients unable to lie flat: learning from the past (letter). *Eye* 2008; 22: 860. DOI:10.1038/sj.eye. 6703032.

[21] Liu C. phacoemulsification in a patient with torticollis (letter). *J Cataract Refract Surg.* 1995; 21: 364.

In: Kyphosis
Editor: Janice Newton

ISBN: 978-1-63483-224-3

Chapter VI

Treatment of Congenital Kyphosis

M. Imtiaz Ghani, MD
Consultant Spine Surgeon, Apollo Group of Hospitals,
Chennai, India

Abstract

Non-Operative Treatments. Observation: Observation is usually the first method of treatment for a young child with a spinal deformity. The visits to the physician will be spaced according to the likelihood of measuring a significant change in the X-ray between each visit. Type I deformities are more likely to have several visits per year. Severe or progressive congenital kyphosis deformities greater than 45° or kyphosis associated with neurologic weakness are usually treated surgically. Early surgical intervention generally produces the best results and can halt progression of the curve. The type of surgical procedure will depend on the nature of the abnormality.

Bracing: Unfortunately, bracing is not recommended when treating congenital scoliosis. Clinical studies fail to demonstrate improved patient outcomes with this method of treatment.

Surgical Treatments. In Situ Fusion: The surgical choice for a progressive kyphotic deformity is a solid fusion or arthrodesis of the deformed vertebrae. The fusion may also include one normal vertebra above and one normal vertebra below this area. Bone graft from the patient or tissue bank is placed posteriorly, on the back of the spine, along the area of the abnormality. In severely angulated curves, additional bone graft may be placed anteriorly, on the front of the spine, as well as from behind. The fusion may be performed with or without the use of instrumentation.

In situ fusion is a non-instrumented fusion without correction of the angulation. The bone graft will require 4-6 months to mature into a solid fusion mass. During the postoperative period the fusion must be protected with a cast or brace until X-rays demonstrate a solid fusion.

Instrumented Fusion and Osteotomy. With progressive kyphotic curves in older children, surgery may include instrumentation (rods, hooks, and screws) that helps to correct the deformity. If the spinal cord is unable to tolerate the manipulative techniques that "straighten" the spine, the surgeon may consider the removal of the mis-shapened vertebrae to realign the spine.

Pedicle subtraction osteotomies and Vertebral column resections are various methods of treatment depending upon severity of deformity and surgeon preference.

Introduction

Kyphosis (from Greek – *kyphos*, a hump), also called *roundback* or *Kelso's hunchback*, is a condition of over-curvature of the thoracic vertebrae (upper back).

A normal thoracic spine extends from the 1st to the 12th vertebra and should have a slight kyphosis ranging from 20° to 45°. When the "roundness" of the upper spine increases past 45° it is called "hyperkyphosis."

While most cases of kyphosis are mild and only require routine monitoring, serious cases can be debilitating. High degrees of kyphosis can cause severe pain and discomfort, breathing and digestion difficulties, cardiovascular irregularities, neurological compromise and, in the more severe cases, significantly shortened life-spans.

These types of high end curves typically do not respond well to conservative treatment, and almost always warrant spinal fusion surgery, which can successfully restore the body's natural degree of curvature. The **Cobb angle** is the preferred method of measuring kyphosis.

Causes

- **Postural kyphosis**, the most common type, normally attributed to slouching, can occur in both the old and the young. In the young, it can be called 'slouching' and is reversible by correcting muscular imbalances. In the old, it may be called 'hyperkyphosis' or 'dowager's hump'. About one third of the most severe hyperkyphosis cases have vertebral fractures. Otherwise, the aging body tends towards a loss of musculoskeletal integrity, and kyphosis can develop due to aging alone.
- **Scheuermann's kyphosis** is significantly worse cosmetically and can cause varying degrees of pain, and can also affect different areas of the spine (the most common being the mid-thoracic area). Scheuermann's disease is considered a form of juvenile osteochondrosis of the spine, and is more commonly called Scheuermann's disease. It is found mostly in teenagers and presents a significantly worse deformity than postural kyphosis. A patient suffering from Scheuermann's kyphosis cannot consciously correct posture. The apex of the curve, located in the thoracic vertebrae, is quite rigid. The patient may feel pain at this apex, which can be aggravated by physical activity and by long periods of standing or sitting. This can have a significantly detrimental effect on their lives, as their level of activity is curbed by their condition; they may feel isolated or uneasy amongst peers if they are children, depending on the level of deformity. Whereas in postural kyphosis, the vertebrae and disks appear normal, in Scheuermann's kyphosis, they are irregular, often herniated, and wedge-shaped over at least three adjacent levels. Fatigue is a very common symptom, most likely because of the intense muscle work that has to be put into standing and/or sitting properly. The condition appears to run in families. Most patients who undergo surgery to correct their kyphosis have Scheuermann's disease.
- **Congenital kyphosis** can result in infants whose spinal column has not developed correctly in the womb. Vertebrae may be malformed or fused together and can cause further progressive kyphosis as the child develops. Surgical treatment may be necessary at a very early stage and can help maintain a normal curve in coordination with consistent follow-ups to monitor changes. However, the decision to carry out the

procedure can be very difficult due to the potential risks to the child. A congenital kyphosis can also suddenly appear in teenage years, more commonly in children with cerebral palsy and other neurological disorders.

- **Nutritional kyphosis** can result from nutritional deficiencies, especially during childhood, such as vitamin D deficiency (producing rickets), which softens bones and results in curving of the spine and limbs under the child's body weight.
- **Gibbus deformity** is a form of structural kyphosis, often a *sequela* to tuberculosis.
- **Post-traumatic kyphosis** can arise from untreated or ineffectively treated vertebral fractures.

Methods of Treatment

Orthosis (Brace)

The Milwaukee brace is one particular body brace that is often used to treat kyphosis in the US. Modern CAD/CAM braces are used in Europe to treat different types of kyphosis. These are much easier to wear and have better in-brace corrections than reported for the Milwaukee brace. Since there are different curve patterns (thoracic, thoracolumbar and lumbar), different types of brace are in use, with different advantages and disadvantages.

Specialised Physical Therapy

In Germany, a standard treatment for both Scheuermann's disease and lumbar kyphosis is the *Schroth method*, a system of physical therapy for scoliosis and related spinal deformities. It involves lying supine, placing a pillow under the scapular region and posteriorly stretching the cervical spine.

Surgery

Surgical treatment can be used in severe cases. In patients with progressive kyphotic deformity due to vertebral collapse, a procedure called a kyphoplasty may arrest the deformity and relieve the pain. Kyphoplasty is a minimally invasive procedure, requiring only a small opening in the skin. The main goal is to return the damaged vertebra as close as possible to its original height.

Treatment of Congenital Kyphosis

Non-Operative Treatments

Observation

Observation is usually the first method of treatment for a young child with a spinal deformity. The visits to the physician will be spaced according to the likelihood of measuring a significant change in the X-ray between each visit. Type I deformities are more likely to have several visits per year. Severe or progressive congenital kyphosis deformities greater than 45° or kyphosis associated with neurologic weakness are usually treated surgically. Early surgical intervention generally produces the best results and can halt progression of the curve. The type of surgical procedure will depend on the nature of the abnormality.

Bracing

Unfortunately, bracing is not recommended when treating congenital scoliosis. Clinical studies fail to demonstrate improved patient outcomes with this method of treatment.

Surgical Treatments

In Situ Fusion

The surgical choice for a progressive kyphotic deformity is a solid fusion or arthrodesis of the deformed vertebrae. The fusion may also include one normal vertebra above and one normal vertebra below this area. Bone graft from the patient or tissue bank is placed posteriorly, on the back of the spine, along the area of the abnormality. In severely angulated curves, additional bone graft may be placed anteriorly, on the front of the spine, as well as from behind. The fusion may be performed with or without the use of instrumentation.

In situ fusion is a non-instrumented fusion without correction of the angulation. The bone graft will require 4-6 months to mature into a solid fusion mass. During the postoperative period the fusion must be protected with a cast or brace until X-rays demonstrate a solid fusion.

Instrumented Fusion and Osteotomy

With progressive kyphotic curves in older children, surgery may include instrumentation (rods, hooks, and screws) that helps to correct the deformity. If the spinal cord is unable to tolerate the manipulative techniques that "straighten" the spine, the surgeon may consider the removal of the mis-shapened vertebrae to realign the spine. The postoperative course remains the same until the fusion mass is determined by X-ray to be solid.

Your surgeon may recommend an osteotomy (bone-cutting procedure) to re-align the spine. Pedicle subtraction osteotomies work by removing the bone in the back of the vertebra so the bone can be collapsed backwards. Vertebral column resections allow resection of the front and the back of the spine from a posterior procedure. The surgeon may also recommend separate approaches from the front and the back of the spine.

Treatment of Developmental Kyphosis

Nonsurgical Management

Observation

Observation is typically recommended in the following situations:

1. Postural hyperkyphosis (their round back straightens with proper posture),
2. Curves that are less than 60° in patients that are growing, or
3. Curves 60°-80° in patients that are done growing.

Standing, long-cassette (scoliosis) X-rays are taken every 6 months as the child grows. If the child has pain, an exercise program is usually recommended.

Bracing

When the deformity is moderately severe (60°-80°) and the patient remains skeletally immature, brace treatment in conjunction with an exercise program is the recommended treatment. Full time use of a brace (20 hours/day) is usually required initially until maximum correction has been achieved. The brace fit must be regularly evaluated and adjusted to ensure optimal correction. During the last year of treatment prior to skeletal maturity, part time brace wear (12-14 hours/day) may be proposed. Brace wear must be continued for a minimum of 18 months in order to maintain a significant, permanent correction of the deformity.

Surgical Treatment

Spinal Fusion

When the kyphotic deformity has become severe (greater than 80o) and the patient is often experiencing increased back pain, surgical treatment may be recommended. Surgical intervention allows significant correction to be achieved typically without the need for postoperative bracing. Pedicle screws are placed (2 per level) and connected with two rods. This process allows gentle straightening of the spine. Most surgeries are performed from the back. However, some physicians recommend additional surgery on the front of the spine. Patients are usually able to return to normal daily activities within 4-6 months following surgery. The correction achieved from surgical intervention is remarkable.

Smith-Peterson (Posterior) Osteotomy

Moderately flexible curves often straighten just from lying prone (face down) on the operating room table. However, rigid curves require additional steps.

The Smith-Peterson osteotomy is often performed at multiple levels to allow safe application of additional corrective forces. Every spinal segment is limited in extension (backward bend) by two sliding facet joints. If these joints are removed, and the disc in front is mobile, approximately 5-10°/level of additional extension is possible to obtain.

Traumatic Kyphosis

Flexible deformities can be treated with posterior fusion and instrumentation. Fixed deformities often require more complex surgery.

Complications

Body Image

Older children with kyphosis may become self-conscious and embarrassed about the effect of kyphosis on their appearance and body image, or the fact that they have to wear a back brace. Anything that makes them 'stand out from the crowd' can be an issue of concern.

This can affect children in different ways and some children may:

a. become socially withdrawn
b. be reluctant to take part in activities that may expose their back or the fact that they have to wear a brace
c. become moodbe reluctant to discuss issues surrounding their treatment, or perhaps argue that they do not need any more treatment

There are no easy answers to these problems, but it can sometimes help to reassure your child that their condition is temporary and will improve with time.

Physical Complications

Other complications of kyphosis usually only occur in more severe cases. They include:

- persistent pain that cannot be controlled with medication
- breathing difficulties that are caused by the spine compressing the lungs and airways

Occasionally, people with kyphosis can have difficulties when the nerves running through the spine become compressed or pinched. This can disrupt nerve signals and cause symptoms such as:

- Numbness or weakness in your arms and legs
- Problems with your sense of balance
- Loss of normal bladder or bowel control (*urinary incontinence and bowel incontinence)*

The risk of serious complications from spinal fusion surgery for kyphosis is estimated to be 5%, similar to the risks of surgery for scoliosis. According to the latest evidence, the actual rate of complications may be substantially higher. Even among those who do not suffer serious complications, 5% of patients require re-operation within five years of the procedure, and in general it is not yet clear what to expect from spine surgery in the long-term. Taking into account that signs and symptoms of spinal deformity cannot be changed by surgical intervention, surgery remains to be a cosmetic indication. Unfortunately, the cosmetic effects of surgery are not necessarily stable. In case one decides to undergo surgery, a specialised centre should be preferred.

Index

C

D

E

F

G

H

I

J

K

L

M

Q

R

S

T

U

V

W

Y